Medical Technolo
and the Social

Medical Technology and the Social

How Medical Technology is Impacting Social Relations, Institutions, and Beliefs About What is Normal

Edited by

Kathryn Burrows

LEXINGTON BOOKS
Lanham • Boulder • New York • London

Published by Lexington Books
An imprint of The Rowman & Littlefield Publishing Group, Inc.
4501 Forbes Boulevard, Suite 200, Lanham, Maryland 20706
www.rowman.com

86-90 Paul Street, London EC2A 4NE

British Library Cataloguing in Publication Information Available

Library of Congress Cataloging-in-Publication Data

Names: Burrows, Kathryn Elizabeth, 1975- editor.
Title: Medical technology and the social : how medical technology is impacting social relations, institutions, and beliefs about what is normal / edited by Kathryn Burrows.
Description: Lanham : Lexington Books, [2024] | Includes bibliographical references and index.
Identifiers: LCCN 2023048925 (print) | LCCN 2023048926 (ebook) | ISBN 9781666940947 (cloth) | ISBN 9781666940954 (ebook)
Subjects: MESH: Biomedical Technology | Social Change | Diffusion of Innovation | Global Health
Classification: LCC R859 (print) | LCC R859 (ebook) | NLM W 82 | DDC 610.285--dc23/eng/20231215
LC record available at https://lccn.loc.gov/2023048925
LC ebook record available at https://lccn.loc.gov/2023048926

Contents

Introduction

Kathryn Burrows

Medical technology is not a product of modernity, as is often assumed: as early as 950 BC, Egyptians were using wooden and leather prosthetics for missing toes (The University of Manchester 2012). For at least 3,000 years, humans have *invented t*ools, devices, and products for the advancement of health, medicine, and wellness. However, we could perhaps date the modern revolution of medical technology to Jenner's invention of vaccines in 1798, the use of surgical lighting beginning in the 1850s, or Roentgen's discovery of X-rays in 1895. More recently, advanced medical technology, such as imaging technology like fMRIs, cochlear implants and other prosthetics, IVF and other reproductive technologies, and, most recently, the use of AI in medicine and surgery, have transformed not only medicine, but also the social world and institutions in which we live. Prenatal ultrasounds now can tell expectant parents the sex of their unborn child, changing the experience of pregnancy; advanced gender-affirming surgery can now be performed altering not only a person's appearance, but their very identity; telehealth has expanded access to healthcare to homebound or rural patients; and 3D printing has enabled the production of customized organs and limbs. In addition to these technologies, advances in pharmacology have allowed some people with profound psychiatric disorders such as schizophrenia to work, have families, and live "normal" lives, and have given people with conditions as diverse as diabetes and ALS a longer life span. And, across all these technological inventions, the question of "what is normal" lingers; is it "normal" to have access to prosthetic blades that can enhance physical performance; is it "normal" to take 15–30 pills a day to manage chronic diseases; is it "normal" to have a pig heart transplanted into a human body?

Medical technologies cannot be separated from "technology" more broadly. After all, even the internet affects bodies in terms of the posture we take when using it, the fingers used to strike keys or swipe left, and the brain waves used to interpret and interact with data. Building technologies affect bodies by the ways structures interact with people's physicality, and even the most advanced space warfare technology ultimately affects bodies by the warfare they rain down on unsuspecting people.

Bronzino, Smith, and Wade (n.d.) wrote one of the first comprehensive manuals about medical technology and society with their *Medical Technology and Society*. The book describes the origins of basic surgical practices and goes up to the modern day (up to 1990) with advanced surgical and medical techniques. Other books and articles soon followed, such as De Miranda, Doggett, and Evans' 2005 article, "Medical Technology: Contexts and Content in Science and Technology," in which they explored the history and impact of medical technology. Ramptom et al. (2022) followed, exploring how the history of medical technology gave rise to the digital technologies of today. The academic discipline of the History of Science, Technology, and Medicine combines the disciplines of the histories of science, technology, and medicine into one mega-discipline that studies the coalescence of all three ("History of Science, Technology and Medicine" n.d.), and is often embedded in larger History of Science and Technology programs.

Society and Medical Technology scholars cover practically every topic covered under the broad umbrella of "society and medical technology" from articles about the history of surgery (Granov 2018; Lirici and Hüscher 2016), to reproductive technologies and race (Seifer, Zackula, and Grainger 2010; Wellons et al. 2012), to prosthetics and gender (Rooker et al. 2019; Straayer 2020) to the scientific processes of medical discovery (Coccia 2014; Gittelman 2016; Wang et al. 2021). Medical technology and society scholars have the wide world of medical technology open to study, and this volume demonstrates this, as scholars in this volume explore everything from fax machines in hospitals to fetal imagery.

This volume is divided into three main sections: Technology Adoption, Diffusion, and Obduracy; Envisioning the Body through Technology; and Pharmaceutical Interventions to the Social World. Papers in each section take a different theoretical and methodological approach, including autoethnography, sociohistorical analysis, and in-depth interviewing, and combine theories of feminist scholarship, STS theory, disability studies, and critical environmental theory.

TECHNOLOGY ADOPTION, DIFFUSION, AND OBDURACY

In "Deconstructing Adoption and Use of Medical Technology: The Case of Two Imaging Technologies in India," Dr. Ankita Mukherjee and Dr. Indira Chakravarthi explore the adoption and diffusion of MRI and CT scanning in India, beginning in the late 1970s. Using the social shaping of technology (SST) and the social construction of technology (SCOT) perspectives, this exploration indicates that the adoption and diffusion of these medical technologies has been a complex process, involving interactions between sections of the medical profession, business, the state, and prevailing social values. They conclude with a brief discussion of the use of fetal ultrasound in India and how it has been used for sex-selective abortions, demonstrating the social power of technology and the intricate weaving between the social and the technological.

In "Infrastructural Embeddedness and the Persistence of Fax in Australian Healthcare Contexts," Dr. Rowan Wilken and Dr. Jenny Kennedy explore the persistence of a so-called "obsolete" technology—the fax machine—in the Australian healthcare setting. They draw on interviews with healthcare and technology professionals spanning a ten-year period. Using technology obduracy theory, they explore the reasons why the fax has persisted in healthcare in Australia. The portrait that emerged from this study is of a complicated socio-technical picture, with manifold, interconnecting framing issues (at different scales) contributing to the continued presence and ongoing embrace of fax machines. The fax persists due to *complexities of everyday data cultures*, where fax has, over years of use, come to constitute a crucial technology and form of health communication technology infrastructure that is well-embedded across the whole healthcare sector. And, the fax persists due to *technological complexities*, as there is a plethora of proprietary, competing encrypted systems on the market that have long had difficulty speaking to each other.

ENVISIONING THE BODY THROUGH TECHNOLOGY

In her autoethnography, "The Fetal Scan Project," Dr. Anna Gonzalez Sucro reconstructs from memory how and why she tried to change the social norm of saving the fetal scan as a keepsake. She worked for pregnant people in exchange for their fetal scan, an object that traditionally has been kept by pregnant people as a memento of their pregnancy. To contextualize her personal story about working with and for the fetal scans of pregnant people as an artist, she engages with feminist debates on reproductive technologies and imagery, which analyze the techno-scientific construction of the fetus through its visualization and medicalization. She situates the artistic use of the fetal scan in a historical context and in relation to socioeconomic factors and political issues.

"The Alterlife of Disabled Fetal Imaginaries" by Dr. Misria Shaik Ali looks at the life of farmers in South India who have been exposed to environmental toxins and irradiation due to uranium mining. Families in the irradiated area have borne children with severe disabilities, or have unwanted childlessness, and Shaik Ali examines how these farmers negotiate disability and reproductive harm in the face of environmental violence. As people become irradiated and their bodies come to bear radiation's effects, she analyzes how the new nuclear and environmental governance model weakens decentralized health governance in the area while strengthening private healthcare.

In "Menstrual Futures: Medical Technologies' Impact on Beliefs about 'Normal' Bleeding," Amber Brooks explores the social meanings of menstruation in the face of menstruation-limiting or suppression technologies, and how menstruation technologies such as hormonal intrauterine devices (IUD) impact the way people who menstruate see themselves and their bodies. She outlines key processes of biomedicalization and Feminist STS perspectives that consider how medical technologies change social relations, institutions, and beliefs about what is normal. She examines evolving menstrual scripts and investigates discourses around the Mirena and Kyleena IUDs, analyzing how new menstrual scripts demonstrate and construct new definitions around menstrual bleeding, and how these discourses produce new subjectivities.

In "The Emporia of Aristotle: What Prosthetics Taught Us About the Human Body," Alan Hawk provides a detailed history of prosthetic lower limbs, including legs, knees, and feet, and while doing so, provides a clear explanation of the human body's posture and gait, and how technologies meant to replace the lower limbs had to adapt to the body's natural gait. He shows how technology is an iterative process and evolves to meet the needs of the human body. He describes how medical authority arose in the discipline, from private inventors to surgeons to prosthetists and explains the relationship between medical devices devised for military purposes that eventually became mainstream technology available to civilians.

PHARMACEUTICAL INTERVENTIONS TO THE SOCIAL WORLD

In "Technologies of Repair: Naloxone, Opioid Overdose Prevention, and the Social in the U.S. Southwest," Dr. Danielle Kabella explores the social implications of naloxone, an emergency medication used in the case of opiate overdose. They show that wider access to take-home-naloxone emerged out of various struggles connected to issues of mass incarceration and premature death. Through its sociomaterial design and spatial entanglements with care it has rearticulated peer and familial social networks by prioritizing connection over isolation giving rise to an alternative collective overdose response and alternate forms of somatic expertise. They argue that the pharmacological effects are optimized through dynamic entanglements of caring practices and relationships that also unsettle drug enforcement, psychotherapeutic approaches and risk environment, and medical authority and expertise.

In "Abilify MyCite and the Social Control of Digital Pills," Dr. Kathryn Burrows explores in a theoretical piece the power and social control elements of the emerging technology of digital pills, focusing on the first digital pill to be approved by the US FDA, Abilify MyCite. She explores issues of medical surveillance and how digital medicine is changing and reinforcing the responsibilities and privileges of people with chronic conditions. The modern notion of responsibility of an ill person is framed in a twofold model: first, protecting other people as part of a public health agenda; and second, as a personal responsibility to one's own health. She examines how digital pills buffer these concepts of responsibility.

REFERENCES

Bronzino, Joseph D., Vincent H. Smith, and Maurice L. Wade. n.d. *Medical Technology and Society*. MIT Press. Accessed May 24, 2023. https://mitpress.mit.edu/9780262521543/medical-technology-and-society/

Coccia, Mario. 2014. "Converging Scientific Fields and New Technological Paradigms as Main Drivers of the Division of Scientific Labour in Drug Discovery Process: The Effects on Strategic Management of the R&D Corporate Change." *Technology Analysis & Strategic Management* 26 (7): 733–49. https://doi.org/10.1080/09537325.2014.882501.

De Miranda, Michael A., Mark Doggett, and Jane T. Evans. 2005. "Medical Technology: Contexts and Content in Science and Technology." Architectural and Manufacturing Sciences Faculty Publications. Paper 5. https://digitalcommons.wku.edu/arch_mfg_fac_pub/5

Gittelman, Michelle. 2016. "The Revolution Re-Visited: Clinical and Genetics Research Paradigms and the Productivity Paradox in Drug Discovery." *Research Policy* 45 (8): 1570–85. https://doi.org/10.1016/j.respol.2016.01.007.

Granov, D. A. 2018. "On the 100-th Anniversary of 'Russian Scientific Center of Radiology and Surgical Technologies Named after A.M. Granov': History of the Development of Surgery." *Вестник Хирургии Имени И.И. Грекова* 177 (5): 94–95. https://doi.org/10.24884/0042-4625-2018-177-5-94-95.

"History of Science, Technology and Medicine." n.d. Accessed May 24, 2023. https://www.ou.edu/admissions/academics/arts-sciences/history-science-tech-med.

Lirici, Marco Maria, and Cristiano G. S. Hüscher. 2016. "Techniques and Technology Evolution of Rectal Cancer Surgery: A History of More than a Hundred Years." *Minimally Invasive Therapy & Allied Technologies* 25 (5): 226–33. https://doi.org/10.1080/13645706.2016.1198381.

Rampton, Vanessa, Maria Böhmer, and Anita Winkler. 2022. "Medical Technologies Past and Present: How History Helps to Understand the Digital Era." *Journal of Medical Humanities* 43 (2): 343–64. https://doi.org/10.1007/s10912-021-09699-x.

Rooker, Steven A., Krishna S. Vyas, Emma C. DiFilippo, Ian T. Nolan, Shane D. Morrison, and Richard A. Santucci. 2019. "The Rise of the Neophallus: A Systematic Review of Penile Prosthetic Outcomes and Complications in Gender-Affirming Surgery." *The Journal of Sexual Medicine* 16 (5): 661–72. https://doi.org/10.1016/j.jsxm.2019.03.009.

Seifer, David B., Rosey Zackula, and David A. Grainger. 2010. "Trends of Racial Disparities in Assisted Reproductive Technology Outcomes in Black Women Compared with White Women: Society for Assisted Reproductive Technology 1999 and 2000 vs. 2004–2006." *Fertility and Sterility* 93 (2): 626–35. https://doi.org/10.1016/j.fertnstert.2009.02.084.

Straayer, Chris. 2020. "Trans Men's Stealth Aesthetics: Navigating Penile Prosthetics and 'Gender Fraud.'" 2020. https://journals-sagepub-com.proxy.lib.pdx.edu/doi/full/10.1177/1470412920946827.

The University of Manchester. 2012. "Egyptian Toes Likely to Be the World's Oldest Prosthetics." http://bit.ly/1Z9Evuh.

Wang, Xuefeng, Shuo Zhang, Yuqin Liu, Jian Du, and Heng Huang. 2021. "How Pharmaceutical Innovation Evolves: The Path from Science to Technological Development to Marketable Drugs." *Technological Forecasting and Social Change* 167 (June): 120698. https://doi.org/10.1016/j.techfore.2021.120698.

Wellons, Melissa F., Victor Y. Fujimoto, Valerie L. Baker, Debbie S. Barrington, Diana Broomfield, William H. Catherino, Gloria Richard-Davis, Mary Ryan, Kim Thornton, and Alicia Y. Armstrong. 2012. "Race Matters: A Systematic Review of Racial/Ethnic Disparity in Society for Assisted Reproductive Technology Reported Outcomes." *Fertility and Sterility* 98 (2): 406–9. https://doi.org/10.1016/j.fertnstert.2012.05.012.

PART I

Technology Adoption, Diffusion, and Obduracy

Chapter 1

Deconstructing Adoption and Use of Medical Technology

The Case of Two Imaging Technologies in India

Ankita Mukherjee and Indira Chakravarthi

Technology has come to occupy a very important status over the past century in what is termed modern or scientific medicine.[1] It is considered an inevitable and desirable feature of modern medical practice and healthcare and argued that there is a technological imperative in medicine (Hoffman 2002). It is less well-known that the introduction and acceptance of medical technologies in modern medicine has been a long, drawn-out process, marked by tensions and contestation between the proponents and opponents of the concerned technology over their efficacy and the place of technology in medicine and public health. In the late nineteenth and early twentieth centuries, by which time technologies like the X-ray and the clinical laboratory had started becoming widespread, important questions arose within the medical profession over the uncritical reliance of medicine on technologically generated facts, over the wisdom of over-reliance on information obtained by technology (Reiser 1978, 171, 173, 183). Within modern medicine and public health, there exist debates and ambivalence about "high technology medicine." To some "it is a milestone marking progress in medicine while to others it is seen as a milestone holding back progress towards an era of preventive and holistic medicine" (Jennett 1983).

The adoption and diffusion of medical technologies have important implications for the quality, safety, accessibility, cost, and affordability of medical care. The presence of regulatory bodies that review and approve medical technologies for clinical use may lead one to assume that medical technologies that have diffused in the health system have been rigorously evaluated and are safe, effective, cost-effective, and better than available alternatives. However, it has been found that adoption and diffusion of medical technologies does not follow a tidy, linear path; factors other than their need, efficacy, and safety shape the adoption and diffusion of medical technologies and strong evidence for their need or effectiveness may not be present before their initial adoption and diffusion (Stocking and Morrison 1978, McKinlay 1981, Banta 1980). This chapter discusses the adoption and diffusion of medical technologies in India, by examining two imaging technologies that were developing around the same time in the 1970s (Blume 1992), the computerized tomographic scanner (CT) and magnetic resonance imaging (MRI). Using primary and secondary sources the chapter explores the processes at the individual, organizational, and societal level that led to the adoption and diffusion of the CT and MRI.

The chapter begins by briefly outlining approaches in technology studies including medical technology. We then describe features of the medical and healthcare system in India to provide the background for the subsequent description and analysis of the diffusion of these technologies in India.

TECHNOLOGY STUDIES

Technological determinism (TD)—the view that technology is autonomous and that it impinges on society from the outside—has been the most influential theory regarding the relationship between technology and society and is the dominant perspective guiding much of the study of technology, including medical technology (de Oliveira 2014, 131; Balconi et al. 2010, 5; Godin 2006, 639). The traditional linear model of technical innovation/development from the TD perspective considers technologies as "applied science," emerging through a sequential flow from basic science research, through applied research and development (R&D) of the technical innovation, to commercial production and use. The research-innovation-diffusion processes are conceived as separate stages in an essentially linear process. The innovations or technical artifacts then diffuse through the marketplace to have impacts upon society.

The social shaping of technology (SST) and the social construction of technology (SCOT) perspectives provide useful critiques of TD and have generated a rich collection of studies on technology and society. Together, they offer insights into the complexity of the process of the development of technology and its role in society, into the social processes of the conception, invention, design, and development of technology, all of which embody particular social relations (Russell and Williams 2002; Williams and Edge 1996; Bijker et al. 1987; MacKenzie and Wajcman 1985, 1999). Research in these genres explores a range of factors—organizational, political, economic, and cultural—which pattern the design and form of technology, as well as the direction of technological innovation. The SST approach has been further extended to look downstream of the social origins of technology innovations. To this end, it has also explored activities such as marketing, at how the technology is implemented or gets used, and appropriation by users. SST studies have examined the commercial shaping of technologies, and suppliers and users of technologies, focusing on areas such as processes of selection, acquisition, and appropriation of technologies in specific contexts; the extent of innovation as technologies diffuse and are used; and the relations and strategies of developers and users in shaping the innovative activity. It is recognized that a range of actors other than manufacturers are involved in the shaping of technology. Users, competing suppliers, and suppliers of complementary products participate in developing markets. Where there is no existing market for a "new technology," the "market" may have to be created to go with the products if suppliers are to realize its commercial potential (Williams 1997). This implies diffusion of the knowledge required to understand the utility of new products and how to use them. So, mapping the industry structures becomes crucial to understanding the shaping of technologies. SST has drawn attention to the close and reciprocal interactions between these stages, and the transformation of technologies between their initial conception and eventual application has helped draw attention to the role of the user and supplier. It has extended its focus "outward" to incorporate analysis of physical and organizational infrastructures, of industrial policies, and of regulation and taxation, among others in shaping technologies.

MEDICAL TECHNOLOGY STUDIES

Since the 1970s medical technology assessment and research have become an independent area of study, a large proportion of which evaluates its impact on the cost of healthcare delivery and on regulatory mechanisms. Such studies have provided useful observations and insights on the diffusion of several medical technologies, including CT scanners (Jennett 1984; Smith 1984; Mechanic 1982; Stocking and Morrison 1978; Office of Technology Assessment 1978). Attention has been drawn to the limitations of classical diffusion theory, which focusses on the role of an individual physician in learning about and then adopting innovations and transmitting information about it (Greer 1982, 272); and the lack of attention to fiscal-managerial organizational issues and political aspects of decision-making in diffusion has been highlighted by several researchers (McKinlay 1982). Greer (1982) drew attention to the potential of Krause's theory (1971) to factor in political aspects of decision making in adoption and diffusion, to Krause's suggestion to examine the role of manufacturing corporations in the promotion of innovations and their coalitions with the interests of physician researchers "to undertake 'frontier research' and others who desired the prestige that had come to be attached to advanced technology" (Greer 1982, 290). Blume's (1992) study comparing the development of the four dominant imaging technologies (X-ray, CT, USG, and MRI) examined the research process by which these technologies took shape—the exploration, development, diffusion, and evaluation—along with the inter-organizational structure between the radiological profession and the manufacturing industry as well as the development of shared interests between sellers and buyers that were vital to the innovation and diffusion of these technologies.

Science, Technology, and Society studies (STS) are a blind spot in India (Visvanathan 2001) and medical technology studies are no exception. While vaccines and pharmaceuticals receive much attention, studies are lacking on medical devices and equipment, on their place in public health, and their diffusion, distribution, access, costs, and impact.

MEDICINE AND HEALTHCARE IN INDIA

In India, modern medicine, also called western medicine or allopathic medicine, became the dominant system over the nineteenth century, and is provided in the public as well as private healthcare sectors. Colonial policies and later the national government's policies after Indian Independence in 1947 ensured the dominance of western medicine from among a plurality of medical practices that existed in the pre-colonial and colonial period (Arnold 1993; Government of India 1946).

Western medical technology diffused into the country in the early years following Independence in a number of ways: through medical education, research, and missions; multinational corporate transactions; technical assistance projects sponsored by the WHO; and bilateral foreign aid programs (Jeffrey 1988). Much of this technology was installed through the state into public institutions and national health programs. A study of the extent to which eight medical techniques, all of which required specific machinery and equipment (ultrasonic fetal examination, fiber-optic endoscopy, cardiac catheterization, renal dialysis, cobalt isotopes for radiotherapy, open heart surgery, CT scanner, and laser beam therapy), had been introduced in some less developed countries by 1977, showed that, except for the CT scanner, all had been introduced in India in government teaching institutions (Piachaud

1977). Another route of diffusion was through non-resident Indian doctors. In the mid-1980s, the American Association of Physicians of Indian Origin (AAPIO), formed in the US in 1982, actively took up projects in India for providing Continuing Medical Education (CME) to Indian doctors and also provided medical equipment to teaching hospitals. The AAPIO, along with the Indian Ministry of Health and the Medical Council of India (MCI), started a scheme to train doctors in Indian hospitals in new technologies (Editorial 1988, 1985). Indian doctors from the US conducted over 150 seminars and "hands-on" courses in over 20 specialties in different institutions across India. Thousands of doctors attended these conferences. The AAPIO also set up a foundation for the donation of used equipment to government hospitals in the country from American members and individual doctors, by which over 100 pieces of major medical equipment, which included CT scanners, dialysis machines, X-ray units, mammography, operating microscopes, and the like, were placed in government hospitals in India.

In the 1980s, the Indian government put in place policies for promoting private investment in the healthcare sector, particularly for specialty and super-specialty services, along with promoting India for investment in the healthcare sector and for low-cost quality medical care (medical tourism). These measures also facilitated the diffusion of medical technologies into the country. The lack of a manufacturing base for advanced medical equipment led to the import of a large amount of equipment and machines that attracted a high customs duty of 150 to 300 percent. This was seen as a barrier to private sector investment; hence the government provided duty exemption to health care institutions for the import of medical equipment (Bhat 2000). There was a steep increase in the variety and sheer volume through the 1990s in the import of medical equipment into the country, including imaging equipment like the CT and MRI (Chakravarthi 2013; Mahal et al. 2006).

Computed tomography (CT) scanners pass X-rays through a body part from different angles to map a structure in two or three dimensions. The CT scanner, developed during the 1960s–1970s, is well known for its extremely rapid diffusion in its initial years, which triggered questions in policy circles in the US and Europe about the costs of technology. The prototype was developed not by the established big X-ray manufacturers then, but by Godfrey Hounsfield from Electric and Musical Industries (EMI) of the UK, a music record label and early manufacturer of gramophones (Blume 1992). This new instrument was announced in 1972 at the 32nd Annual Congress of the British Institute of Radiology and the same year at the Radiological Society of North America (RSNA) meeting. The images produced by the scanner created quite a sensation and soon a huge and enthusiastic demand for it arose from the medical profession. The potential threat posed by a development like the CT scanner by an outside firm such as EMI to the existing medical

X-ray manufacturers forced them to respond, leading to intense competition and a rapid rate of technical change; CT scanners soon became big business. By the end of 1975 there were at least twenty firms that had developed or were developing CT scanners. One of the key features which impacted the diffusion of the technology was the rapid innovation cycle and the consequent changes in the CT scanner. The early head scanner developed by Hounsfield in 1972, also called first-generation scanners, gave way to faster full body second-generation scanners in 1975 which reduced the scan time by almost half. Third-generation scanners were on the market by 1978.

CT SCANNERS COME TO INDIA: THE EARLY ADOPTERS

Dr. Sneh Bhargava, a radiologist from the All-India Institute of Medical Sciences (AIIMS), India's premier leading medical institution in New Delhi, was present at the historic 1972 RSNA meeting where Hounsfield showed his images. She recalls that he got a standing ovation from the audience after his presentation. As to her reaction, she said, "I obviously understood that this is going to change the whole face of diagnostic related radiology and the practice of medicine." Dr. Bhargava explained how Hounsfield's adaptation was ingenious, as for the first time, cross-sectional images could be obtained:

> The human body is a three-dimensional body. And you could only record one dimension [using X-rays]. . . . So, he [Hounsfield] came out with the technology by which the X-ray was made to rotate around the body. If you have a loaf of bread, you see a loaf of bread, when you do an X-ray, you get the image of the loaf of bread. But his technology sliced the loaf. So that at every slice, you could produce an image.

On returning from this conference, Dr. Bhargava requested that the director of AIIMS procure a CT scanner instead of a new X-ray that she had been demanding. A team from AIIMS therefore made several requests to the health ministry. This was a time when the private corporate healthcare sector was beginning to make its presence in India's tertiary healthcare sector. AIIMS was the foremost teaching and research hospital in the country and was often the first institution to which the government allotted funds for adopting newer technologies. However, one CT scanner cost about Rs 45 lakhs (about 1.4 million USD today), which was a prohibitively large sum for a piece of equipment at that time. The government therefore was reluctant to fund the equipment. It was the Swedish bilateral agency, the Swedish International Development Cooperation Agency (SIDA), which eventually funded the equipment as well as provided training. Radiologists from AIIMS, including Dr. Bhargava, were sent to the Karolinska Institute to learn about CT scanning. AIIMS finally obtained its first head scanner in April 1978 from the General Electric Company (GEC), in England. In the five years that it took for arranging for funds and constructing the building to house the CT, the technology had undergone rapid change. By 1978 the third-generation full body scanners had already entered the market in the US.

Although the head scanner at AIIMS did provide the first exposure for neurologists as well as radiologists to the CT scanner, access to the education and medical facilities at AIIMS was limited. The spread of a technology like the CT scanner depended on information and knowledge about this technology among more sections of medical professionals. In the late 1970s and early 1980s, Indian radiologists were not trained in using the CT. Doctors from AIIMS did publish and present information about the scanner. Had AIIMS remained the only institution to have the technology for another couple of years, only a few radiologists would have been able to get hands-on experience and training in this new modality and the diffusion would have been much slower. However, this was not the case. By the early 1980s, India would see many (perhaps hundreds of) radiologists, including those in smaller towns, interacting with the technology, many of whom would go on to start their own imaging businesses and become established names in the field of radio-diagnosis. Private diagnostic companies, such as Medinova Diagnostics of Hyderabad, Surlux Diagnostic Centre Ltd. Bombay, and United Group, were setting up diagnostic centers in many parts of the country offering CT scanning. The United Group is credited with importing and setting up the first brain scanner in India in the private sector in 1980. Within a decade, by 1990, India was reported to have around 100 body scanners; cities like Bombay (now Mumbai) had 13 body scanners, Delhi 11, and Madras (now Chennai) had 8 (Jesani and Anantharam). The man responsible for this was a Delhi-based businessman, R. K. Gupta, who started the United Group in the early 1980s. Several radiologists who were interviewed for this paper mentioned the role that Gupta's United Group played in the diffusion of the technology in the early 1980s.

Mr. Gupta was running a successful construction business when he entered the imaging business by chance. An airplane encounter with a person who was going to the US to get a brain scan using a new technology triggered Gupta to explore the possibility of providing this new technology in India. R. K Gupta had little knowledge of the medical field or about the market for such services. He credited his late friend and neighbor Dr. Arjun Dev Sehgal, a then well-known neurosurgeon who had trained at the Cleveland Clinic in the US, for motivating him. Dr. Sehgal had headed neurological departments in leading public and private hospitals in Delhi, was president of the Neurological Society of India, and held other important positions in the specialty. He also established the Sehgal Neurological Research Institute in New Delhi in 1969 (Delhi Neurological Association) and incorporated ADS Diagnostics Limited in 1984 for trading, installing, and servicing medical equipment in India.

Gupta acquired the first CT scanner from a little-known California-based company, Omni Medical, with help from Dr. Sehgal's brother in California. According to one of the radiologists interviewed, the equipment Gupta imported was "rudimentary." Two other radiologists mentioned that these were secondhand scanners. While the exact specifications of the equipment that Gupta imported were not available, he was the first in the private sector (at least in Delhi and perhaps the whole country) to install a head scanner. The scanner was first installed in 1980 at his home in Kailash Colony. Early patients came from Dr. Sehgal's nursing home and as the word spread more patients were referred. Mr. Gupta recalls that they were doing up to ten scans a day, at a cost of Rs 1000 (about USD 273 today) per scan.

As the imaging business progressed, Gupta started importing parts from Omni Medical, assembled and installed them in imaging centers owned by him across the country. Mr. Gupta recalls that there were about 30 centers across the country. In these centers radiologists who had no prior interaction with the technology started learning about its application through hands-on work. In the words of a renowned radiologist from Delhi:

> So, it was this Mr RK Gupta who in the beginning got (the CT), and there were several other businessmen like him. Doctors had no intention or thoughts of becoming entrepreneurs. Those were the era of stability in life, get a job and make merry. But Mr. Gupta needs to be credited as far as CT goes, for bringing that technology into the country.
>
> —Senior Radiologist (KI05)

Later, Gupta partnered with Toshiba to import and assemble full body scanners. But the business was faltering by then as bigger players had entered the Indian market. Eventually Gupta had to close his imaging business in the early 1990s as he felt that the centers were being mismanaged and there was swindling of money by local staff, leading to losses.

Although several radiologist respondents acknowledged the role of R. K Gupta in early diffusion of the technology, at least in two instances, there was a perception that his business was not entirely transparent. One radiologist mentioned:

> He used his contacts in the government to get the deal and obviously it was completely fraudulent in the sense that he over invoiced, made a lot of money

> out of this. . . . But what he did was responsible for the amazing growth of CT scanning in India because an entire generation of radiologists were employed in his centers and they all became extremely good radiologists as time went by because they learnt. And CT scan services were available in 50 cities in India, at one go.
>
> —Senior Radiologist (KI03)

Mr. Gupta, however, reiterated that he "tried to serve the cause of the people" through his business.

Dr. Arjun Dev Sehgal eventually disengaged with R. K. Gupta (Sehgal's son indicated that it was over financial matters). But by this time Dr. Sehgal had decided to continue to be involved in the business of imaging. This time he partnered with another of his neighbors and a patient, Vipin Singal, a businessman who operated a tours and travel company at the time. Vipin Singal could not be contacted for this study, and therefore information about his partnership with Arjun Dev Sehgal was provided by Gautam Sehgal, son of Arjun Dev Sehgal. Arjun Dev Sehgal became the director and promoter of Vipin Singal's company, SNS Pharma, which procured and installed the first modern third-generation whole-body CT scanner at a leading private hospital in Delhi—Sir Gangaram Hospital in 1982–1983. Arjun Dev Sehgal was a senior consultant in the hospital and played an important role in facilitating the process. SNS Pharma was responsible for providing the equipment as well as radiologists who would do the scans. Sehgal received a share of the income generated from the business. Two senior radiologists who had worked with SNS Pharma recalled the installation of the full body CT scanner at Sir Gangaram Hospital as a watershed moment for CT imaging. While the scanner at AIIMS and Gupta's head scanners gave medical professionals the first exposure to the technology, it was the scanner at Gangaram which signalled the broader diffusion of the technology. This can be attributed to the major advancements in the technology that had taken place by then. Scanning times had been reduced significantly, image quality had improved, and a whole-body scanner meant specialists other than neurosurgeons could now explore the application of the technology. According to one radiologist who worked on the first scanner at Gangaram,

> CT became available at AIIMS in 1979. But that was only a head scanner. And it had its utility, and it could work for only a sub-segment of patients related to radiology and neurosurgery. But in the year '82 there was an explosion of CT technology when it became available for whole body imaging. We were

> the first to have it in Sir Gangaram Hospital in December 1982 and it became operational in January 1983.
>
> —Senior Radiologist (KI04)

He further recalled how the experience was truly transformative for him and for the whole field of medicine:

> We were really thrilled with the reality of [what you could get]. It's not possible to explain that in 5–10 minutes. There are hundreds of examples. People used to think that in pancreatitis there would be no free fluid but now we see fluid in every alternate patient, appendix we can diagnose so easily, brain tumors we could diagnose so easily [. . .] . We were struggling earlier for years together, for decades together. It totally revealed the details of the body.
>
> —Senior Radiologist (KI04)

Eventually the relationship between SNS Pharma and Dr. Sehgal disintegrated because of matters of financial irregularity. In the past he had disengaged with Gupta over similar concerns. It is possible that due to failure of his two partnership ventures, he chose to start a company of his own. Arjun Dev Sehgal then started ADS Diagnostics, which started several imaging centers in and around Delhi, where CT scanning and subsequently MRI too were made available. SNS Pharma had to close its diagnostic imaging business. According to Gautam Sehgal, his father was the real force behind popularizing the model of private imaging center chains in North India and gained much respect in the field of neurosurgery for popularizing new CT-based interventions and uses of CT diagnosis in conditions like epilepsy.

MAGNETIC RESONANCE IMAGING (MRI): INVENTION, MARKETING AND EARLY DIFFUSION

The MRI machine is a large magnet with a hollow bore surrounded by coils which send radiofrequency pulses. Humans are placed inside the bore of the magnet and exposed to radiofrequency pulses. The hydrogen atoms in our body are exposed to a magnetic field and then to specific radiofrequency pulses. Due to a phenomenon known as *nuclear magnetic resonance*,[2] the hydrogen nuclei emit a radiofrequency pulse which is captured by a computer connected to the MRI. These signals are interpreted and transformed into images.

Raymond Damadian, a physician at Downstate Medical Center in New York, produced the first MRI machine for human imaging in 1977. However, it is Paul Lauterber, a chemistry professor with research experience in Nuclear Magnetic Resonance (NMR) and chairman of the NMR Specialities Corporation, who is credited with developing the technique to be used in clinical settings. Several other teams in the US and UK were also involved in the research and development of the MRI (Blume 1992; Prasad 2014) Many of the prominent scientists involved in early research and development of the MRI collaborated with industry players in the early commercialization of the technology, and by the early 1980s, most major manufacturers had started clinical placement of their machines.

The MRI had a very different trajectory of diffusion compared to the CT scanner. For the CT scanner, the market and clinical application were clear from the very beginning. In fact, the medical fraternity, especially neurologists, was waiting eagerly to get their hands on the machine. The case of MRI was not the same. There was neither a clear idea of the exact use or market for the equipment or its advantages over the CT scanner. Even issues like whether a permanent or superconducting magnet was to be used or in which department in the hospital it should be placed were not clear (Hillman and Goldsmith 2011).

The centrality of the US healthcare market in the development of expensive technologies needs to be noted. US healthcare has traditionally been more profitable and has been culturally amenable to adopting new technologies. In Prasad's (2014) words this "celebratory embrace of hi-tech medicine" led to acceptance of MRI in the US even when its full uses were not clear. It was also prohibitively expensive and installation costs were high. Safety concerns also existed as the long-term impact of radiofrequency heating on tissues was not completely known (Prasad 2014). In the early 1980s most of the studies assessing safety were still animal studies (McRobbie and Foster 1985a; McRobbie and Foster 1985b; Schwarz and Crooks 1982). Nevertheless, the MRI was (and still is) considered a much safer modality than the CT scanner as the latter uses ionizing X-ray radiation while the former uses radiofrequency waves. Despite these uncertainties, the MRI was already represented as a medical marvel in popular literature in America since its early days. Another implication of the primacy of the US market was the change of name from "Nuclear" Magnetic Resonance to Magnetic Resonance Imaging. The word *nuclear* was dropped by manufacturers because of the negative association of radiation with the term *nuclear* among the American public. There were popular protests and movements against nuclear power plants and nuclear weapons at the time and there were concerns about harms from radiation. People did not trust that MRI was safe and did not use radiation, and resisted installation of these machines in their neighborhood healthcare facilities. The term Magnetic Resonance Imaging was therefore promoted by American physicians and hospital administrators (Kelly 2006).

Much of the demand in the early years was from research institutions who purchased the equipment at relatively lower rates than the clinical price. Manufacturers who needed clinical data in order to receive FDA approval were eager to place units in such institutions (Hillman and Schwartz 1985). By 1984, the advantages of NMR imaging for the brain and central nervous system were beginning to be recognized and the potential for imaging other organs was still being explored. By August of 1984, there were 145 NMR imagers in clinical settings across the globe, out of which 93, or 64 percent, were located in the United States. This was a steep increase from January 1983 when only 14 units had been installed in the US (Office of Technology Assessment 1984). The US Congress, Office of Technology Assessment Report on NMR imaging noted:

> [Moreover]despite the rapid improvement in the quality of NMR images that has occurred over the past several years and the increasingly large number of clinical situations in which NMR imaging might prove to be of value, the exact role of NMR imaging in clinical medicine, particularly its efficacy compared to other imaging modalities, has yet to be defined. (Office of Technology Assessment 1984, OTA-HCS-27, p. 3)

Commercial marketing of MRIs began in 1985. The popularity of the MRI in this phase was more due to its *potential* rather than proven evidence about its utility over other modalities or a full understanding of its clinical uses. Since then, the uses of MRI have expanded, and it has found its place in modern medicine.

THE MRI COMES TO INDIA: STORY OF THE EARLY ADOPTERS

The first MRI was installed in India in 1986 at the Institute of Nuclear Medicine and Allied Sciences (INMAS), a research laboratory of the government Defence Research and Development Organisation (DRDO) in Delhi. Its director, Major General N. Lakshmipathy, is credited with bringing the MRI to the Institute. Lakshmipathy's associates, who were part of the team who worked on India's first MRI machine, remember him as a "visionary" and a "genius" who went out of his way to get exciting new technology to India. The early research team at INMAS consisted of two doctors, Amar Nath Jena (nuclear medicine) and Rakesh Kumar Gupta (radiology), along with physicist Subhash Khushu and several other technical staff to support the running of the equipment (Prasad 2006).

Major General Lakshmipathy resolved to bring an MRI to INMAS after viewing the in-vivo images shared by a British scientist, at a conference at INMAS around 1982–1983. At that time, MRI research had not established its complete clinical application nor its advantages over existing modalities (most notably the CT scanner). In the 1980s the MRI was "rudimentary," and many of the sequences[3] required for imaging started coming in from 1987. Yet in 1984, Lakshmipathy was already travelling to the US, the UK, and Germany to obtain information about the MRI.

There were two kinds of responses from Lakshmipathy's associates about his motivations for bringing an extremely expensive technology to INMAS, the clinical uses of which were still being researched. The first reason cited was that he was a visionary who was able to think like other great minds of world in anticipating its possible benefits.

> In [19]80s, MRI was rudimentary. . . . Looking at the images that were then available, it was very difficult to assess its usefulness. At that time, he conceived [that] perhaps it has got a biological use back home, where it is going to help in better diagnosis. Or, he must have been in sync with what the other people were thinking elsewhere in the world. There was no demand or compulsion that we should get an MRI into the health system because it is doing something marvellous. But here it is a different story. That means somebody thought it is to be good in the future, so he conceived the idea and worked relentlessly . . . [to get the technology].
>
> —Senior Radiologist (KI17)

It is difficult to know if Lakshmipathy had anticipated that one day the MRI would become an integral part of clinical diagnostic medicine. According to one of his associates, Lakshmipathy had not known about cross-sectional imaging, instead he saw MRI as useful for nuclear medicine. Amit Prasad (2006) reiterates this and mentions that Lakshmipathy had envisioned MRI to be part of a "panel of nuclear medicine." He had not envisioned its application in the field of radiology for cross-sectional imaging, which is the most common application of the MRI today.

There is another opinion regarding Lakshmipathy's motivations which does credit him as being a visionary but attributes more pragmatic reasons to his decision to acquire the MRI. In discussing what may have motivated Lakshmipathy to acquire the MRI, one of his associates felt that it was likely that Lakshmipathy had found something "that could make or break the institution" and getting the MRI would be "another feather in his cap." The prestige associated with acquiring the technology for Lakshmipathy personally as well as for INMAS are hinted at by his associate. It must, however, be remembered that INMAS is primarily a government research institution, therefore it could justify acquiring a technology for undertaking further research.

Whatever the motivation for Major General Lakshmipathy was, he did work relentlessly to import the equipment. Apart from travelling to international centers to learn more about the technology, he also made close associations with leading names in nuclear medicine and imaging research like Henry Wagner of Johns Hopkins and Leon Partain and Everett James of Vanderbilt University. Exposure to works of leading researchers in the field may have contributed to shaping his desire to acquire an MRI. One of the major concerns for Lakshmipathy was the cost of the project. Apart from the exorbitant cost of the equipment itself, installation and maintenance costs were also going to be prohibitive. A multidisciplinary team of engineers, nuclear physicists, and specialists in nuclear medicine and radiology were needed. INMAS had acquired a 1.5 tesla[4] superconducting magnet[5] which had further implications for cost. Liquid helium, which is used for cooling the superconducting magnet, had to be imported. Two things worked in favor of INMAS when it came to these cost prohibitions. The first was that it was a defense establishment, which meant it had access to a larger budget than other institutions, such as those that were under the health department. One can assume that many questions would have been raised if a public hospital had hoped to acquire the technology at this stage. Secondly, Lakshmipathy's association with the then prime minister of India, Rajiv Gandhi, ensured that cost would not be a barrier to get the technology to India and that he would not face any bureaucratic hurdles in his endeavor (Prasad 2006). INMAS was one of the premier institutions which provided medical services to key government functionaries at the time, and this had helped Lakshmipathy to cultivate contacts with the prime minister. He was assured all financial assistance to procure MRI for INMAS. Eventually Siemens was engaged through a turnkey project for the equipment and installation. A liquid helium and nitrogen plant was set up inside INMAS to ensure uninterrupted supply.

It is difficult to know the exact cost of the whole project between equipment and installation costs, and different sources give different estimates. According to Dr. R. K. Gupta, the project cost about INR 60 million (USD 10.5 million today). Amit Prasad, who interviewed Lakshmipathy, mentions a figure of INR 80 million (USD 14 million today) (Prasad 2006). A representative from Siemens who was involved in the project at the time estimated that the entire project may have cost INR 150–200 million (USD 26–35 million today)—although it seems an overestimate compared to what the others have quoted.

Dr. Jena, an associate of Lakshmipathy recalls that getting the equipment from the airport to INMAS was nothing short of a ceremony. There was fear that bad roads may damage the equipment during its transportation. Major

General Lakshmipathy collaborated with the Public Works Department to ensure that the MRI had a smooth ride to INMAS. The MRI at INMAS became operational in 1987 at its Centre of Nuclear Magnetic Resonance.

The early reaction from the medical fraternity was understandably guarded. Dr. Gupta mentions that several reputed radiologists, including those from AIIMS, visited their center but were not enamored with the technology especially given its cost. Dr. Jena said, "In 1985–86 everyone was on the fence-line, whether it (MRI) is going to work or whether it is going to fail." Admittedly, the challenges to establish and operate the equipment were huge. In fact, the uncertainty about the capability of the MRI was so great that when R. K. Gupta joined the MRI research team at INMAS, his senior colleagues felt that he had committed "professional suicide." These early scientists did not have much research to rely on, and interpreting images was not easy.

Becoming an early adopter of the technology and being a research institution helped INMAS to anchor much of the early research and later diffusion of MRI expertise, especially in, though not restricted to, Delhi. Many of the prominent radiologists who built up expertise in the early decade of the technology trained at INMAS. Some, like R. K. Gupta, subsequently went to the public sector at the Sanjay Gandhi Post Graduate Institute, Lucknow, and undertook MRI research. Others started their own private imaging centers. Viral Shah, a radiologist who had trained at Beth Israel Hospital in New York, is credited with getting the first MRI in the private sector installed in 1987 at Bombay's Breach Candy Hospital (Prasad 2006) almost at the same time as at INMAS. Shah had also been involved with MRI clinical research during his stint at Beth Israel. The private sector in Delhi started to adopt the technology in the early 1990s, with independent radiologist-owned centers like Mahajan Imaging and Diwanchand Aggarwal Imaging installing the MRI.

In these initial years, when awareness about these technologies was limited among the medical fraternity and medical colleges did not teach about these new modalities, many doctors learned through hands-on training. The huge investment that equipment like the CT and MRI required could only be recovered if an effective demand for the service was created, which was only possible through information dissemination among the medical fraternity about advantages of using these modalities. In the case of the CT scanner, acceptance of the technology was easy because of the relative advantage over existing techniques. One of the doctors associated with Sir Gangaram Hospital at the time says, "We were the first people [to use CT scanners]. Very quickly within 2–3 months we were travelling all over the country, giving lectures [about application of MRI] in front of whole medical colleges" (Senior Radiologist [KI04]). When the MRI entered the market, there was intense debate over its uses and advantages over the CT scanner, not the least because it was extremely expensive. One early adopter of the MRI recounts how one of the biggest challenges was to educate doctors about the new modality,

> I went around the country giving lectures on MRI. And the first slide used to be advantages of MRI over CT. So, it was a huge task. When we started, we wouldn't do even five cases a day.
>
> —Senior Radiologist (KI05)

These early radiologists also therefore became advocates of the technology among the medical fraternity.

MEDICAL TECHNOLOGY DIFFUSION: EXPLANATIONS AND IMPLICATIONS

In this section we discuss how diffusion of medical technology is not just a function of technology itself or its perceived utility, but rather its interactions with individuals, institutions, markets, society, and the state within which it is embedded. We also explore some of the current implications of diffusion of medical technologies using examples of CT and MRI and substantiate our arguments using some other examples like ultrasonography.

INDIVIDUALS, INSTITUTIONS, PREROGATIVES

The cases of the CT and the MRI demonstrate that certain individuals take the lead in adoption and diffusion of new technologies. They may be motivated by the relative advantages of the technology or, in the absence of evidence, by the estimated potential of the technology. These individuals are often located in institutions where resources and networks enable them to procure the innovations and undergo training in their use. Access to networks and resources is key. In the cases of the CT and MRI scanners it was determined individuals, located in different types of institutional settings, public and private, who played a significant role in facilitating adoption of these technologies. There are both similarities and differences in the stories of these early sites of technology adoption. In both cases, the lead was taken by physicians in the public sector who had trained in or had exposure and access to knowledge networks in the medical system in the US or UK. The position and access to international networks for these physicians conferred advantages and prestige that enabled their access to financial resources to procure these technologies for their institutions. With Dr. Bhargava's presence, AIIMS was able to convince the Ministry of Health to direct funds from a grant by SIDA to buy a

CT scanner and arrange for the training. The informal links of Major General Lakshmipathy with the then prime minister was critical to getting funds for the MRI at INMAS.

In the private sector, at least in Delhi, we see collaboration between physicians and local businessmen. In the case of the CT, two businessmen made early investments to provide CT services in the private sector. However, both partnered with a reputed neurosurgeon trained at Cleveland Clinic, who had knowledge and exposure to benefits of the technology and could refer patients. For early adopters in the private sector the stakes were very high. In the 1980s when CT scanners started coming in, import duties were extremely high and interest rates were anywhere between 24 and 27 percent. Costs were therefore prohibitive. Local businessmen did not have knowledge of the diagnostic imaging field and while physicians had the technical knowledge, they lacked financial resources to import the technology. It is for this reason that in many cases, we see a collaboration between radiologists and businesspersons through which both benefitted.

Decision making regarding early technology adoption is governed largely by institutional factors such as resource availability. We find a clear distinction between priorities and decision making in public and private medical facilities. For publicly funded medical or research institutions, the key decision makers are senior physicians of the concerned department. Decisions are made often through departmental consensus. Therefore, the kind of technology that is acquired depends on how well physicians are exposed to current research and advancements. In private corporate hospitals the top-level management plays an important role in identifying new technologies that need to be acquired. Concerned physicians too may raise a demand for novel technologies, bringing new technologies to the notice of the management. But big-ticket technologies such as the CT and MRI were often the decisions of the top management.

There is a difference in the way costs and benefits are evaluated in publicly funded and privately owned institutions. In public hospitals there are clear bidding guidelines for procurement (as per General Financial Rules), which must be abided by, and any proposal has to pass through several hierarchies for approval. In the government sector, cost is the most important variable. The bidding process is designed in a manner that the least expensive item which satisfies the minimum requirement wins the bid. In the private sector cost is only a secondary consideration. While public institutions must justify their need for an equipment based on expected utilization, in the private sector, utilization and the need to be "at par with whatever is happening in the market" are factored in. There is of course a clear cost-recovery strategy, which means that when an expensive technology like CT or MRI is upgraded, the "volumes generated" in the hospital become a crucial consideration. This has important implications for patients. As hospitals must work on generating volumes (attracting more patients) to recover costs of technology like the CT or MRI, it creates a field ripe for potential conflict of interest. As one senior radiologist pointed out:

> See there would be a little possibility that whenever somebody invests in technology, the particular investor would be keen to see that he gets back his return on investment. Now whether you call that pressure or whether you call that expectation and how that works in different environments is very variable. So I have heard stories that I believe there are many people who have invested so they are very keen to push doctors to generate that kind of a return by asking for many investigations.
>
> —Senior Specialist, private hospital (KI21)

Doctors who were interviewed for the study were categorical in denying such practices as setting of targets by management in hospitals in which they practiced. However, some studies mention instances of hospitals setting investigation targets for doctors, leading to unnecessary investigations (Marathe et al. 2020; Gadre and Shukla 2016, 3–32). Unnecessary investigations have been widely reported for over a decade now. Many doctors have been expressing concern and drawing attention to the practice of overdiagnosis or excessive investigations and the associated practice of offering commissions (or "cuts") to doctors for diagnostic investigation referrals to private imaging centers (Berger 2014). In 2013 Dr. Himmatrao Bawaskar returned a check that was sent to him by a private diagnostic center with branches in the cities of Mumbai and Pune, towards "professional fee for referring a patient to their center for MRI" (Bawaskar 2013, 278); he also filed a complaint against the diagnostic center with the Medical Council of India (Sachan 2013). Following this, it was no longer possible for doctors to deny that this practice was prevalent. In 2014 cardiologists at AIIMS, Delhi, launched an initiative called the Society for Less Investigative Medicine (SLIM), to tackle the increasing practice of advising excessive medical investigations (Nagarajan 2015). In 2017 doctors at a conference on the nature of healthcare at Tata Memorial Hospital, Mumbai, pointed out that around 30 percent of medical tests and high-tech applications, including MRIs and ultrasounds conducted in a private healthcare setup, were completely irrelevant and only increased the patient's medical bill by thousands of rupees; according to them, when a private hospital invested resources in procuring a technology, it was under pressure to recover the cost and the only way to do so was to prescribe more scans, whether or not they were indicated medically (Mukherjee 2017). Such practices by doctors and private diagnostic centers or hospitals, to recover costs of technology, have implications for cost of care, which is primarily borne by patients in India from personal finances (out-of-pocket expenditure). There are also safety implications due to exposure to X-radiation in the case of the CT scanner, where patients may be exposed to unnecessary radiation.

TECHNOLOGY AND THE MARKET

In their early phases, these technologies went through rapid innovation cycles. Often these expensive technologies became obsolete within a few years of acquisition. This was quite apparent in the case of the CT scanner. Between 1972 and 1978, EMI had already moved from head scanners to producing third-generation CT whole-body scanners. It was similar for MRI. An executive from Siemens who was interviewed recalled that in the 1990s, innovation cycles were only four or five years.

Radiologists who adopt a new or improved version of technology often become an important source of dissemination of information about these technologies. Interestingly, the owners of a new technology take up the role of marketing the advantages of their equipment within the radiology community.

> We also go and disseminate information in our clinical meetings and conferences and show beautiful images done on a three tesla and some of the procedures that we do only on a three tesla. For example, if I am one of the early birds to buy a 3-tesla unit would I not try to disseminate it in the profession?
>
> —Senior Radiologist (KI07)

While early adopters became important advocates of the technology, manufacturers of these technologies played and continue to play an equally important role in its diffusion. The arrival of these technologies in the late 1980s to early 1990s coincided with economic liberalization policies in India, and led to increased private sector participation in healthcare, and the emergence of an affluent, aspirational class with ability to pay for healthcare. In other words, the emergence of a huge healthcare market held many opportunities for growth and profits for the Indian healthcare industry, which encompassed the medical equipment industry. The latter started engaging in activities beyond manufacture and trade; in intense promotion of their technologies, in the financing, supplying peripherals, customer advice, and education, and in healthcare delivery as well. The multinational equipment manufacturers give wide publicity each time any of what are portrayed as "advanced equipment"/"breakthrough technology"/"revolutionary technology" was installed in any healthcare facility. To give just one example: GE announced prominently the installation of its LightSpeed Volume CT scanner (VCT) at Jaslok Hospital in Mumbai in October 2005 (General Electric 2005) and a 16-slice CT scanner capable of providing PET-CT scans,[6] as "the first such system in India," at Tata Memorial Hospital in Mumbai in December 2004 (Pharmabiz Bureau 2004). As education and training in these imaging modalities was not yet part of the medical curriculum, multinational imaging manufacturers such as GE, Philips, and Siemens started organizing education, training, and research in medical imaging and trials in academic centers, to complement manufacturing and trading. Continuing medical education courses, seminars, conferences, product launches at medical conferences, demonstrations of ultrasound scanning on live subjects, and exhibitions of medical equipment, all sponsored and funded by the equipment industry, were the major means of acquiring and exchanging information about new technologies and procedures. They also started consulting with hospitals and clinics on ways to procure, or lease and finance, their purchases. For example, Siemens partnered with a bank for financing purchases of its medical equipment (Chakravarthi 2013). The issue of industry influence on physician decisions regarding technology and that of conflict of interest in the above arrangements of the industry with the hospital and/or diagnostic center, and the subject of regulation of diagnostic technologies, such as imaging technologies, have not received much scholarly attention (Hogarth et al. 2022).

Opening up of the economy paved the way for private equity investment in healthcare in a number of corporate hospitals (Chakravarthi et al. 2023). This shift in the very nature of ownership of tertiary health care providers (from mostly government-owned tertiary hospitals to expansion in private equity–funded corporate hospitals) has also been responsible for rapid diffusion of expensive and high-end novel medical technologies including more advanced CT and MRI variants. Due to the very nature of these for-profit business enterprises, their distribution is skewed towards the profitable tertiary care sector with most hospitals operating as super-specialty or multispecialty hospitals in resource-rich urban centers. Super-speciality hospitals have to make significant investment in cutting-edge technology. The competition ensures that every corporate hospital presents (advertises) itself as equipped with state-of-the-art technology. One senior physician observed how the private sector in India has taken the lead in getting novel technologies:

> So once upon a time, I think when we were doing our training, so I think the government hospitals were always the ones which had the latest technology. So the best ultrasounds and CTs came to All India Institute of Medical Sciences (AIIMS) and private sector was not at all at par. They were way behind. For whatever reasons, over the last 15–20 years, it is the private sector which seems to be getting the technology early, and the latest technology, whereas it is not

> often coming to the government sector, it's coming late. In a way that is what has made a whole lot of aspiring patients come to the private hospitals. So good or bad I will leave that to your judgement or anybody's judgement, but that is the phenomenon.
>
> —Senior Specialist, private hospital (KI21)

This has implications for the health system. As competition among the private super- speciality hospitals grows, there is increasing pressure to invest in high-end novel technologies that serve as a differentiator. Getting a return on these investments for these hospitals (which are essentially business enterprises) becomes crucial and keeps pushing up marketing expenses, all of which contributes to cost of care.

MEDICAL TECHNOLOGY AND SOCIETY

Technologies, including medical technologies, both are shaped by and shape society. The diffusion of imaging technologies with increasing complexity and cost shaped the medical profession and perceived disciplinary hierarchies within the medical profession. Nothing demonstrates the primacy of technology in transforming hierarchies in medicine better than the emergence of radiology as a leading branch of medicine in the past three decades. Radiologists repeatedly emphasized the role that technologies like the CT and MRI played in transformation of the field of radiology.

> When I did my post-graduation in 1977, we only had conventional X-ray technology and our training and specialization revolved around plain X-ray. But turn of 1979-80-81, a lot of change came about. Technologically we took a complete leap you know. So this completely changed the way radiology was practiced.
>
> —Senior Radiologist (KI07)

The reputation and glamor associated with radiology has increased as a result of advanced technology and it has come to be regarded as a field that is at the cutting edge and constantly evolving. This has made it one of the most sought-after specializations for medical graduates.

In India radiology was hardly a popular choice for medical graduates till the 1980s. A number of radiologists mentioned that their choice of radiology was not conscious. In fact, there was largely the perception that radiology was for those who could not get a better option to specialize in. As one radiologist put it,

> Radiology was not an upcoming specialty at that time (in the 1980s). Only back benchers used to join the radiology. No one used to join because radiology was just X-ray and nothing else and some investigation with contrast media. In the '80s anyone who has joined radiology, there used to be only two categories, either they are highly fascinated by radiology or they don't have good academic record.
>
> —Senior Radiologist (KI02)

Hillman and Goldsmith (2011) discuss a similar trend in the context of US medicine where until a few decades ago, radiology did not enjoy the venerated place that it has in medicine today. It was technology that helped this relatively obscure specialty to move up "medicine's food chain" (Hillman and Goldsmith 2011). It was the development and integration of high-end diagnostic imaging technologies like the CT and the MRI that started the transformation of the field and indeed the way medicine was practiced. It is a reflection of how "technocentricism" shapes the hierarchy of expertise within the field of medicine. The eighties was a transformative time for medicine. As one radiologist puts it,

> I am extremely fortunate that the day I entered radiology, some sort of technological explosion started happening. Radiology became one of the first and foremost branch.
>
> —Senior Radiologist (KI04)

Slowly but steadily the technological armor at the disposal of radiologists has expanded. Today, along with X-ray machines, a radiologist can use ultrasonography, mammography, DEXA scans, and CT and MRI scanners to obtain images of the human body. Development of PET-CT and PET-MRI have given impetus to the field of nuclear medicine. With the development of advanced imaging techniques, radiologists have now found a role in therapeutic intervention too. Interventional radiology is a field where image guidance through available techniques like CT and MRI is used to assist actual therapeutic intervention (like insertion of a stent). As a result of these changes, the reputation and glamour associated with radiology has increased and it has come to be regarded as a field that is at the cutting edge and constantly evolving. This has made it one of the most sought-after specializations for medical graduates. Other specialties like community medicine have been relegated as non-glamorous even though in a country like India there is significant relevance for these specializations. According to one senior radiologist, although the field has become extremely popular among medical graduates, much of this has to do with the glamour of high-end technology and unrealistic expectation about monetary returns.

> It's probably been a glamorous thing. Students and interns, when they think of radiology, they think of you know these glitzy machines and computers and interventional radiology and stuff like that. It's popular because of all this.
>
> —Senior Radiologist (KI03)

The above example shows how technology diffusion shaped an entire profession. It is also important to highlight that medical technology diffusion can also be shaped by society and its impact on society may be well beyond anticipated medical benefits. Nothing demonstrates this better than the example of ultrasonography (USG) in India. While the chapter primarily uses the example of the CT and the MRI to make its argument, the case of the USG has been discussed because it provides a unique insight into how society and medical technology may interact.

Ultrasonography is a diagnostic imaging modality that is widely used for fetal monitoring during pregnancy and is an important tool for ensuring a safe pregnancy. The case of the diffusion and use of the ultrasound in India illustrates how social norms shaped the use of a technology for purposes it had not been intended for. In India USG has been widely used for the non-medical purpose of sex determination followed by abortion in the case of female fetuses (what has been also termed female feticide).

Patriarchal values have led to a deep-rooted preference for sons, who are seen as potential breadwinners and taking forward the family lineage. In certain religions only males/sons can perform the funeral rites of parents. Daughters, on the other hand, are considered to be like temporary guests who would move to their actual households after marriage. Marriage of girls is a very expensive proposition with the expectation of a dowry from the groom's family and cultural expectations related to lavish weddings. It is not uncommon for families to fall into debt to get their daughters married as the typical cost of a wedding may be several times the annual income of a family. Open advertisements of amniocentesis and ultrasonography with the tagline "Pay Rs 500 now to save Rs 500,000 later," referring to the economic burden of a dowry and other expenses of marrying off daughters, have been reported (Kusum 2000). While some of this could explain son preference among poorer families or among communities with strongly entrenched patriarchal norms, the phenomenon of sex-selective abortions has taken place in India among all sectors, rich and poor, rural and urban, educated and non-educated (Bhalotra and Cochrane 2010). This indicates a more deep-rooted traditionally inherited value system which values boys over girls even though there may be no immediate financial compulsion.

Being non-invasive and less expensive than amniocentesis, as well as the arrival of portable machines, contributed to this spread. With increasing availability of ultrasound, sex determination and sex-selective abortions became more widespread (Oomman and Ganatra 2002). Mobile sex-selection clinics in smaller towns of Haryana state, offering ultrasound detection and immediate abortion if the fetus was female, were also reported in the mid-1980s (Chakravarthi and Hunter 2019). Within a few years of their introduction in the 1980s, tens of thousands of ultrasound scanners were reportedly sold throughout India, with a disproportionate number in northwest India, to medical professionals and possibly also to untrained informal providers (Madan and Breuning 2014). States in the northwest region of India have traditionally had strong patriarchal norms (like gender segregation, veiling or *purdah*, and limited mobility for women) and son preference. The increased availability of ultrasound technology in the prevalent patriarchal context of deep-rooted son preference has been shown to be associated with increased prevalence of prenatal sex selection in several parts of North India, severely affecting the sex ratio at birth (Akbukut-Yuksel and Rosenblum 2022). It is estimated that between 1987 and 2016, about 13.5 million female births were "missing" and this could be attributed to sex-selective abortions. About half the world's missing female births occur in India as a result of sex-selective abortions (Saikia 2021). The implications of a skewed sex ratio are still being understood. In the state of Haryana, which has one of the worst sex ratios, poor women from other states are being brought in as brides often in exchange for money (Roy, Rai, and Nangia 2018).

All medical technologies for prenatal genetic testing or fetal imaging require qualified, trained medical and laboratory staff and expensive equipment. Such large-scale prenatal sex determination would not be possible without the participation and knowledge of medical professionals. Hence the role of medical professionals—the primary users of these technologies—in its adoption, diffusion, and non-medical use, and in mediating its meaning to the lay seekers of such technologies, cannot be ignored. Sections of the medical profession in India have actively enabled, encouraged, and promoted the use of ultrasonography (and amniocentesis) for sex-selective abortions and female feticide (Madan and Breuning 2014; Sharma, Gupta, and Relhan 2007). Offering these technologies became extremely lucrative; doctors, alone or in partnership with wealthy people, took advantage of the deep-rooted patriarchal values of son preference and discrimination against girls in India to set up private USG imaging centers. In the process, they also reinforced patriarchal values and gender discrimination in shaping the meaning of these technologies for lay people.

MEDICAL TECHNOLOGY AND THE STATE

The state plays a crucial role in medical technology diffusion and its use through regulations and legislation as well as shaping broader policies regarding the economy and healthcare sector. The diffusion of the imaging technologies discussed happened in the context of a liberalized economy and expansion of the private medical sector in India. This helped in the diffusion of CT and MRI particularly in the private sector.

Regulation, or the absence of it, has had important implications for the diffusion and adoption of medical technologies. Most medical device regulatory bodies regulate the manufacture and sale of devices and focus on ensuring safety and efficacy. Legislations and oversight over how the technology is utilized by the medical sector is often left to self-regulation.

The manufacture, import, and sale of medical devices in India are overseen by the Central Drugs Standard Control Organisation (CDSCO). Until 2018 there was no comprehensive legislation for medical devices in India. In the absence of comprehensive legislation for medical device regulation, in 2005 the government passed a notification in which some high-risk devices came under the ambit of regulation under the Drugs and Cosmetics Act (DCA), 1940. The manufacture, import, and sale of these "notified devices"[7] required procuring a license and submission of necessary documentation.

Imaging modalities which use radioactive substances or emit ionizing radiation are regulated by the Atomic Energy Regulatory Board (AERB). The AERB is the primary agency responsible for regulating nuclear facilities and use of radioactive materials, which includes industrial as well as medical uses. Nuclear medical devices therefore are regulated under the Atomic Energy Act, 1962. However, radiation-emitting imaging devices came under its purview as late as 2004 after the Atomic Energy (Radiation Protection) Rules, 2004 were promulgated. In the seventies and eighties when the CT and MRI entered the market, there was essentially no substantive regulation covering these two devices.

In the 1970s the medical fraternity was swept off its feet by the potential of new and emerging imaging technologies, propelled by the promise of solutions that technology could offer. Some of these technologies were adopted long before sufficient evidence on their efficacy, safety, and clinical indications was available. Early studies on the effectiveness of new imaging technologies and their safety were quite small and were extremely uncritical (Creditor and Garrett 1977). The safety of these new technologies had not gotten the attention that it should have in a profession associated with healing and health. In the case of CT scanning no attention was paid to radiation dosage levels delivered to the patients, especially to children, despite prior knowledge and experience of the hazards of X-rays. Only with the tremendous increase in CT usage, concerns about the long-term consequences of such exposures started to be addressed, nearly a decade and a half later.

Regulation of misuse of technology or medical malpractice associated with medical technologies is nearly nonexistent in India. The only exception is the nationwide legislation in 1994 that banned sex-selective abortions with provisions for penalties as well as imprisonment for violators. Today every clinic that possesses ultrasonography or other imaging equipment must have a public notice posted that mentions prenatal disclosure of sex is prohibited under law. As discussed, medical practitioners were deeply involved in the practice of using ultrasonography for sex-selective abortions. In the 1990s doctors had indicated that despite bans, they would communicate verbally the sex of the fetus to parents who wanted to know and would hike the test fees to compensate for the legal risk (Sudha and Rajan 1999). This highlights the limitations of self-regulation and state regulation of the ineffectiveness of professional codes of ethics as well as legal instruments, in the face of promising economic gains. Although there have been criticisms about weak implementation and its possible ineffectiveness (Tabaie 2014), others have demonstrated that the policy has achieved some success (Nandi and Deolalikar 2013).

We find diffusion and use of imaging technologies like the CT, MRI, and USG happened in a context of limited regulatory oversight by the state. However, broader policy changes and shifts in the economy and subsequent growth of private sector medical care impacted the diffusion of these technologies.

DISCUSSION AND CONCLUSION

It is important to view medical technology innovation-adoption-diffusion as a dynamic network of relationships among the medical profession–industry-state and patients-users, embedded in and influenced by society, as the SST and SCOT approaches have shown. The story of early adopters of CT and MRI technology demonstrates interactions between individual, organizational, and broader contextual factors leading to adoption and diffusion of these technologies. Individuals could be motivated by the potential of the technologies to improve care or for the associated reputation that they brought. In the public sector, these technologies were acquired by individuals who were associated with institutions of repute, and who could leverage formal and informal networks to acquire the technology. In the case of private individuals, leveraging informal networks and gaining support of champions from the medical fraternity was important.

While individuals and their attributes may play a role, these individuals must be placed within their broader socioeconomic context. Entry of the CT and MRI in the Indian market coincided with important shifts in the economy which in turn transformed the healthcare service sector in India. With economic liberalization and inflow of capital to the private healthcare sector through establishment of super-specialty corporate hospitals and diagnostic service chains, diffusion of the technologies got a boost.

Lastly, the policy-legal framework of the state in shaping diffusion of medical technologies in general should also not be lost sight of. In the Indian context, it was the absence of any substantive regulation for medical devices which shaped the diffusion of these technologies without any regulatory barrier. While cost of these technologies may have been a barrier, the shift in the economy and infusion of private capital into the medical care sector was an important facilitator.

The implications of diffusion of these medical technologies are wide-ranging. Diffusion of expensive imaging technologies in the unregulated private healthcare sector has led to conflict of interest in the medical profession and interests of patients being compromised. Maximizing gains and moving ahead of competition are at the core of many for-profit healthcare providers. For large corporate hospitals and independent imaging centers this means continually investing in state-of-the-art technology. Expensive technologies like the CT and MRI require massive investments and institutions are under pressure to recover costs by acquiring higher patient volumes. This may be done by providing patient number targets to doctors practicing in hospitals. Independent imaging centers often provide commissions to prescribing doctors for sending in patients (Gadre and Shukla 2016). There is clear incentive for physicians to send more patients, even when tests may not be required. Since much of healthcare expenses in India are borne out of pocket, this has financial implications for patients. In the case of the CT, there are health implications as patients may be exposed to unnecessary radiation. Another aspect of the market is the push by manufacturers to sell their products using various means like sponsoring conferences, continuing education, or trainings for doctors. This can impact objective decision-making by doctors who may disregard patient interest in favor of acquiring a technology.

Explanations such as improving medical care and patient welfare, or faith and fascination with the potential of technologies, although not entirely misplaced or unsubstantiated, do not adequately explain the uncritical adoption and diffusion of expensive technologies, especially without evidence of safety, effectiveness, or comparative advantage over existing less expensive technologies. The stepping in of technology manufacturers and other businesses to support these economic concerns, as a component of their promotional activities, are elements that cannot be ignored. Marketing strategies adopted by manufacturers like sponsorship of continuing education of doctors or of conferences are common and open to conflict of interest.

The transformation of the field of radiology demonstrates another implication of diffusion of technologies like CT and MRI. The technological imperative in healthcare (Hoffman 2002), which associates technology with progress and medical technologies with superior healthcare, transformed radiology—which garnered little interest among medical graduates—to one of the most glamorous and sought-after specializations. The value and prestige associated with technology, and the radiologist's ability to manipulate high-end technologies and interpret images, adds to the glamor and prestige associated with radiology as a field of practice within medicine.

The impact of technology can be far more wide-ranging on society. Ultrasonography in India presents a unique example of this. The absence of regulatory oversight, unethical drive for profits by practitioners, and the existing social milieu which prefers sons over daughters together led to unprecedented demographic changes and a skewed sex ratio in favor of males. The implications of this are already being felt in some places with men not finding brides. Long-term implications are yet to be fully understood.

In this chapter we attempted to explain some of the reasons which led to early adoption and diffusion of medical technologies, using the example of the CT and MRI and some of the consequences of diffusion of these technologies. These are closely linked to how markets, society, and the state interact with these technologies.

NOTES

1. There are different systems of healing and medicine in different parts of the world; however, what is widely practiced and is the dominant form for more than a century now is what is termed scientific medicine or modern medicine, which largely developed in European countries and North America. This system of modern medicine became hegemonic and marginalized existing systems of medicine in many countries, such as in India, in the course of their colonization by the British. India had and continues to have several indigenous systems such as Ayurveda, Unani, Siddha. However, it is modern medicine that is the dominant system. The scope and focus of this article are restricted to technology in the current, dominant system of modern medicine.

2. The nuclei of certain atoms like hydrogen have a unique characteristic, in that, if they are placed in a magnetic field they start to align themselves to the magnetic field and move at a particular frequency. When a radio wave is passed through them at these specific frequencies, they tend to absorb that energy and release that energy when returning to their relaxed state once the radio wave is terminated. This phenomenon is known is nuclear magnetic resonance.

Table 1.1.

Annexure

Informant ID	*Age*	*Sex*	*Spcialization*	*Type of Institution associated with*	*Current Position*
KI01	53	Male	Radiology	Private /Stand-alone imaging center	Owner of imaging center & Ex IRIA[8] president
KI02	58	Male	Radiology	Private /Stand-alone imaging center	Owner of imaging center & Ex IRIA president
KI03	52	Male	Radiology	Private /Stand-alone imaging center	Owner of imaging center & Ex IRIA president
KI04	61	Male	Radiology	Private /Stand-alone imaging center	Owner of imaging center & Ex IRIA president
KI05	57	Male	Radiology	Private /Stand-alone imaging center	Owner of imaging center & Ex IRIA president
KI06	29	Male		Private /Stand-alone imaging center	Co-owner of imaging center
KI07	65	Male	Radiology	Private /Stand-alone imaging center	Consultant in different private setups
KI8	37	Male	Radiology	Public/ Superspeciality teaching hospital	Associate Professor
KI9	57	Female	Radiology	Public/ Teaching hospital	Professor
KI10	50	Female	Radiology	Public/ Teaching hospital	Assistant Professor
KI11	51	Male	Radiology	Public/ Superspeciality teaching hospital	Professor
KI12	45	Female	Radiology	Private/ Superspeciality hospital	Senior Consultant

KI13	86	Female	Radiology	Private/Cancer Hospital	Senior Consultant and head of department
KI14	47	Male	Radiology	Private/ Superspeciality hospital	Senior Consultant
KI15	85	Male	Civil engineering		Retired businessman
KI16	57	Male		Company supplying medical equipment	Managing Director
KI17	69	Male	Nuclear Medicine	Private/ Superspeciality hospital	Senior Consultant
KI18	65	Male	Radiology	Private/ Superspeciality hospital	Director and head of department
KI19	41	Male	Hospital Administration	Private /Superspeciality Corporate Hospital	Part of procurement division
KI20	51	Male	Electronics	Siemens	
KI21	61	Male	Gastroenterology	Private/ Superspeciality hospital	Executive Director (of department)

3. MRI sequence refers to technical information on ways to operate the MRI to obtain specific kinds of images.

4. Tesla is a unit which measures magnetic field strength. Today 3 tesla MRIs are available and considered extremely powerful. In the 1980s 1.5 tesla strength was the highest strength available.

5. Magnets used in MRIs can be permanent magnets or superconducting magnets. The former is less powerful (have lower magnetic field strength) and less expensive compared to the latter. Superconducting magnets produce magnetic field by passing electricity through superconducting coils wrapped around them. The temperature of these coils needs to be controlled and kept below a certain temperature. For this, coolants like liquid nitrogen and helium are used.

6. PET-CT or Positron Emission Tomography scans are done on CT scanners. A radioactive tracer is injected in the body which collects on specific tumors and tissues and can be seen during the scan.

7. Notified Devices include Cardiac Stents, Drug Eluding Stents, Catheters, Intra Ocular Lenses, I.V. Cannula, Bone Cements, Heart Valves, Scalp Vein Set, Orthopaedic Implants, Internal Prosthetic Replacements, Disposable Hypodermic Syringes, Disposable Hypodermic Needles, Disposable Perfusion Sets, InVitro diagnostic devices for HIV, HBsAg, and HCV. Other devices regulated as “drugs” are Blood Grouping Sera, Ligatures, Sutures and Staples, Intra Uterine Devices, Condoms, Tubal Rings, Surgical Dressings, Umblical Tapes, and Blood/Blood Component bags.

8. Indian Radiological and Imaging Association (IRIA).

REFERENCES

Akbulut-Yuksel, Mevlude and Daniel Rosenblum. 2002. *Estimating the Effects of Expanding Ultrasound Use on Sex Selection in India*. IZA Institute of Labor Economics, Discussion Paper. IZA DP No. 15838. ISSN: 2365–9793.

Arnold, David. 1993. *Colonizing the Body: State Medicine and Epidemic Disease in Nineteenth-Century India.* Delhi: Oxford University Press.

Balconi, Margherita, Stefano Brusoni, and Luigi Orsenigo. 2010. "In defence of the linear model: An essay." *Research Policy* 39:1–13. DOI:10.1016/j.respol.2009.09.013.

Banta, David H. 1980. "The diffusion of the computed tomography (CT) scanner in the United States." *International Journal of Social Determinants of Health and Health Services* 10(2): 251–69. https://doi.org/10.2190/6D17-3UAU-RAM1-NVTR

Bawaskar, Himmatrao S. 2013. "The Medical Trade." *Indian Journal of Medical Ethics* 10(4): 278. October-December.

Berger, David. 2014. "Corruption ruins the doctor-patient relationship in India." *British Medical Journal* 348. DOI: https://doi.org/10.1136/bmj.g3169 (published May 8, 2014).

Bhalotra, Sonia R. and Tom Cochrane. 2010. *Where Have All the Young Girls Gone? Identification of Sex Selection in India*. IZA Discussion Paper No. 5381. Available at SSRN: https://ssrn.com/abstract=1731185 or http://dx.doi.org/10.2139/ssrn.1731185

Bhat, Ramesh. 2000. "Initiatives to invite private capital through public-private partnerships in social sectors: Some experiences from the health sector." *Vikalpa: The Journal for Decision Makers* 25(3): 37–48. https://doi.org/10.1177/0256090920000305

Bijker, Wiebe E., Thomas P. Hughes, and Trevor Pinch. 1987. *The Social Construction of Technological Systems: New Directions in the Sociology and History of Technology.* Cambridge, Massachusetts: The MIT Press.

Blume, Stuart S. 1992. *Insight and Industry: On the Dynamics of Technological Change in Medicine*. Cambridge, Massachusetts: The MIT Press.

Chakravarthi, Indira. 2013. "Medical Equipment Industry in India: Production, Procurement and Utilization." *Indian Journal of Public Health* 57(4): 203–7.

Chakravarthi, Indira and Benjamin Hunter, eds. 2019. *Regulation of formal private healthcare providers in Maharashtra: Journey of Pre-Conception and Pre-Natal Diagnostics Techniques (Prohibition of Sex Selection) Act, 1994.* Pune: SATHI. Available at: https://unsettlinghealthcare.org/projects/corporatisation-and-regulation/

Chakravarthi, Indira, Shweta Marathe, Benjamin Hunter, and Susan Murray. 2023. "Corporatisation in private hospitals sector in India: Case study from Maharashtra." *Economic & Political Weekly* 58(11): 57–64.

Creditor, Morton C. and Julie B. Garrett. 1977. "The Information Base for Diffusion Of Technology: Computed Tomography Scanning." *New England Journal of Medicine* 297(1): 49–52. DOI: 10.1056/NEJM197707072970110

Delhi Neurological Association. https://dnadelhi.in/dr-arjun-dev-sehgal-oration-2/. Accessed on Feb. 7, 2023.

de Oliveira, Marcos Barbosa. 2014. "Technology and basic science: the linear model of innovation." *Scientle studia*, São Paulo, 12 (special issue): 129–46.

Editorial. 1988. "Market for Outdated Technology." *Economic and Political Weekly* 23(35): 1773. https://www.epw.in/journal/1988/35/uncategorised/health-market-outdated-technology.html

Editorial. 1985. "Medical Technology: Dubious Gift." *Economic and Political Weekly* 20(38): 1580–81.

Gadre, Arun and Abhay Shukla. 2016. *Dissenting Diagnosis.* India: Random House.

Gelijns, Annetine C. and Nathan Rosenberg.1994. "The Dynamics of Technological Change in Medicine." *Health Affairs* 13(3): 28–46.

General Electric Press Release. 2005. "Next-generation GE LightSpeed Volume CT, built on life-saving technology, now in India." September 21. Available at: https://www.ge.com/news/press-releases/next-generation-ge-lightspeed-volume-ct-built-life-saving-technology-now-india. Last accessed May 9, 2023.

Godin, Benoît. 2006. "The Linear Model of Innovation: The Historical Construction of an Analytical Framework." *Science, Technology, & Human Values* 31(6): 639–67. https://doi.org/10.1177/016224390629186

Government of India. 1946. *Report of the Health Survey and Development Committee Vol II: Recommendations*. Delhi: Manager of Publications.

Greer, Ann L. 1982. "Advances in the Study of Diffusion of Innovation in Health Care Organisations." In *Technology and Future of Health Care*: Milbank Reader 8. Edited by John B. McKinlay, 271–98. Cambridge, Massachusetts: The MIT Press.

Hillman, Allan L. and J. Sanford Schwartz. 1986. "The diffusion of MRI: Patterns of siting and ownership in an era of changing incentives." *American Journal of Roentgenology* 146(5): 963–69.

Hillman, Bruce J. and Jeff Charles Goldsmith. 2011. *The Sorcerer's Apprentice: How Medical Imaging Is Changing Health Care*. Oxford University Press, p. 39.

Hoffman, B. 2002. "Is there a technological imperative in healthcare?" *International Journal of Technology Assessment in Health Care* 18(3): 675–89.

Hogarth, Stuart, Fiona Miller, and Steve Sturdy. 2022. Multidisciplinary perspectives on regulation of diagnostic technologies. *Social Science and Medicine* 304: 115059. https://doi.org/10.1016/j.socscimed.2022.115059

Jeffrey, Roger. 1988. *The Politics of Health in India*. Berkeley: University of California Press.

Jennett, Bryan. 1984. *High technology medicine: Benefits and burdens.* London: Nuffield Provincial Hospital Trust.

Jesani, Amar and Saraswathi Anantharam. 1993. *Private sector and Privatisation in the Health Care Services.* Review Paper for the ICSSR-ICMR Joint Panel on Health, August 1990, p. 81. The Foundation for Research in Community Health (FRCH), Bombay. Available at: https://fmesinstitute.org/wp-content/uploads/2022/04/Private-sector-Privatisation1.pdf

Joyce, Kelly A. 2006. "From Numbers to Pictures: The Development of Magnetic Resonance Imaging and the Visual Turn in Medicine." *Science as Culture* Vol. 15, No. 1: 1–22. https://doi.org/10.1080/09505430600639322

Krause, E. A. 1971. "Health and the Politics of Technology." *Inquiry* 8: 51–59.

Kusum, K. 2000. "Sex Selection in India: Case Study." In *Women's Rights and Bioethics*, edited by Lorraine Dennerstein, 52. UNESCO Publishing.

MacKenzie, Donald and Judy Wajcman, eds. 1985. *The Social Shaping of Technology: How the Refrigerator Got Its Hum.* Milton Keynes, UK; Philadelphia: Open University Press.

MacKenzie, Donald and Judy Wajcman. 1999. "Introductory Essay: The Social Shaping of Technology." In *The Social Shaping of Technology*, edited by Donald MacKenzie and Judy Wajcman, 2nd ed. Buckingham: Open University Press.

Madan, Kamlesh and Martijn H. Breuning. 2014. "Impact of prenatal technologies on the sex ratio in India: An overview." *Genetics in Medicine* 16(6): 425–32. DOI: 10.1038/gim.2013.172

Mahal, Ajay, Anil K. Varshney, and Srinicas Taman. 2006. "Diffusion of diagnostic medical devices and policy implications for India." *International Journal of Technology Assessment in Health Care* 22(2): 184–90. DOI: 10.1017/S0266462306051002

Marathe, S., Benjamin Hunter, Indira Chakravarthi, Abhay Shukla, and Susan Murray. 2020. "The impacts of corporatisation of healthcare on medical practice and professionals in Maharashtra, India." *BMJ Global Health* 5: e002026. DOI:10.1136/bmjgh-2019-002026

McKinlay, John B. 1982. "From 'Promising Report' to 'Standard Procedure': Seven Stages in the Career of a Medical Innovation." In *Technology and Future of Health Care*: Milbank Reader 8. Edited by John B. McKinlay, 233–70. Cambridge, Massachusetts: The MIT Press.

McRobbie, D. and M. A. Foster. 1985. "Pulsed Magnetic Field Exposure during Pregnancy and Implications for NMR Foetal Imaging: A Study with Mice." *Magnetic Resonance Imaging* 3(3): 231–34.

Mechanic, David. 1982. "The Growth of Medical Technology and Bureaucracy: Implications for Medical Care." In *Technology and the Future of Health Care*, edited by John B. McKinlay. Milbank Reader 8. Cambridge, Massachusetts: The MIT Press.

Mukherjee, Rupali. 2017. "30% tests by private hospitals are irrelevant, say doctors at meet." *The Times of India*. January 28, 2017. https://timesofindia.indiatimes.com/city/mumbai/30-tests-by-private-hospitals-are-irrelevant-say-doctors-at-meet/articleshow/56819843.cms

Mukherjee, Sonali. 2013. "Skewed Sex Ratio and Migrant Brides in Haryana: Reflections from the Field." *Social Change*, 43(1): 37–52. https://doi.org/10.1177/0049085713475725

Nagarajan, Rema. 2015. Doctors across India join hands to stop practice of unwanted tests. *The Times of India*. May 17, 2015. https://timesofindia.indiatimes.com/india/doctors-across-india-join-hands-to-stop-practice-of-unwanted-tests/articleshow/47313607.cms

Nandi, Arindam, and Anil B. Deolalikar. 2013. "Does a legal ban on sex-selective abortions improve child sex ratios? Evidence from a policy change in India." Journal of Development Economics 103(C): 216–28. DOI: 10.1016/j.jdeveco.2013.02.007

Office of Technology Assessment. 1984. *Health Technology Case Study 27: Nuclear Magnetic Resonance Imaging Technology: A Clinical, Industrial, and Policy Analysis*. U.S. Office of Technology Assessment, Washington, DC. OTA-HCS-27, p. 3.

Office of Technology Assessment. 1978. *Policy Implications of the Computed Tomography (CT) Scanner.* U.S. Congress, Office of Technology Assessment.

Oomman, Nandini and Bela R. Ganatra. 2002. "The Systematic Elimination of Girls." *Reproductive Health Matters* 10(19): 184–88. DOI: 10.1016/S0968-8080(02)00029-0

Pharmabiz Bureau. 2004. "India's first PET/CT system launched at Tata Memorial Hospital." Available at: http://test.pharmabiz.com/news/india-s-first-pet-ct-system-launched-at-tata-memorial-hospital-25234

Piachaud, D. 1979. "The Diffusion of Medical Techniques to Less Developed Countries." *International Journal of Health Services* 9(4): 629–43. DOI: 10.2190/QVK8-J638-W8V7-6F9J

Prasad, Amit. 2006. "Social Adoption of a Technology: Magnetic Resonance Imaging (MRI) in India." *International Journal of Contemporary Sociology* 43: 327–35.

Prasad, Amit. 2014. *Imperial Technoscience: Transnational Histories of MRI in the United States, Britain, and India*. MIT Press.

Reiser, Stanley J. 1978. *Medicine and the Reign of Technology*. Cambridge University Press.

Roy, Archana K., Ambarish K. Rai, and Parveen Nangia. 2018. "Skewed sex ratio, male marriage squeeze and cross-cultural marriages: A study of an ecologically vulnerable region in India." *Canadian Journal of Tropical Geography/Revue canadienne de géographie tropicale*. Vol. 5, No. 2. December 25, 2018, pp. 16–24. URL: http://laurentian.ca/cjtg

Russell, Stewart, and Robin Williams. 2002. "Social shaping of technology: Frameworks, findings and implications for policy with glossary of social shaping concepts." In *Shaping Technology, Guiding Policy: Concepts, Spaces and Tools*, edited by K. H. Sørensen and Robin Williams, 37–132. Cheltenham, UK: Edward Elgar.

Sachan, Dinsa. 2013. "Tackling corruption in Indian medicine." *The Lancet* 382(9905): E23–E24, November 16. DOI: https://doi.org/10.1016/S0140-6736(13)62364-8

Saikia, Nandita, Catherine Meh, Usha Ram, Jayanta Kumar Bora, Bhaskar Mishra, Shailaja Chandra, and Prabhat Jha. 2021. "Trends in missing females at birth in India from 1981 to 2016: Analyses of 2.1 million birth histories in nationally representative surveys." *The Lancet Global Health* 9(6): e813–e821.

Schwartz, J. L. and L. E. Crooks. 1982. "NMR Imaging Produces No Observable Mutations or Cytotoxicity in Mammalian Cells." *American Journal of Roentgenology* 139(3): 583–85. DOI: 10.2214/ajr.139.3.583

Sharma B. R., N. Gupta, and Nidhi Ralhan. 2007. "Misuse of prenatal diagnostic technology for sex-selected abortions and its consequences in India." *Public Health* 121: 854–60. DOI: 10.1016/j.puhe.2007.03.004

Stocking, Barbara and Stuart L. Morrison. 1978. *The image and the reality: A case-study of the impacts of medical technology*. Published for the Nuffield Provincial Hospitals Trust by the Oxford University Press.

Stocking, Barbara, ed. 1988. *Expensive Health Technologies: Regulatory and Administrative Mechanisms in Europe*. Oxford: Oxford University Press.

Sudha, S. and Irudaya Rajan. 1999. "Female Demographic Disadvantage in India 1981–1991: Sex Selective Abortions and Female Infanticide." *Development and Change* 30(3): 585–618. https://doi.org/10.1111/1467-7660.00130

Tabaie, Sheida. 2013. "Stopping female feticide in India: The failure and unintended consequence of ultrasound restriction." *Journal of Global Health* 7(1). DOI: 10.7189/jogh.07.010304

Vishvanathan, Shiv. 2001. "Democracy, Governance and Science: Strange case of the missing discipline." *Economic and Political Weekly* 36(39): 3684–88.

Williams, Robin and David Edge. 1996. "The Social Shaping of Technology." *Research Policy* 25: 865–99. DOI: 10.1016/0048-7333(96)00885-2

Williams, Robin. 1997. "The Social Shaping of Information and Communication Technologies." In *The Social Shaping of Information Superhighways: European and American Roads to the Information Society*, edited by Herbert Kubicek, William Dutton, and Robin Williams, 299–338. Frankfurt; New York: Campus Verlag; St Martin's.

Chapter 2

Infrastructural Embeddedness and the Persistence of Fax in Australian Healthcare Contexts

Rowan Wilken and Jenny Kennedy

In 2018, the Royal College of Surgeons England submitted freedom of information requests to NHS [National Health Service] Trusts on their use of fax machines. These requests revealed that facsimile machines—faxes—formed the "backbone" of NHS communications, with over 9,000 machines still in active use (Kerr 2020). The then UK Health Secretary responded swiftly to this revelation, placing an embargo on the purchase of new fax machines, and launching a campaign to "axe the fax" (Kerr 2020).

In Australia, the focus of this chapter, there have been similar calls to break with the reliance on fax machines as a key communication technology in the healthcare field. For instance, in 2019, the then CEO of the Consumers Health Forum of Australia, Leanne Wells, declared that "manila folders of paper and fax machines aren't good enough in the twenty-first century" (cited in digitalhealth.gov.au 2019). Concern was also raised within the Australian Capital Territory (ACT) government's budget estimates hearings over the continued reliance on faxes within ACT health services (Scott 2019).

This is not just due to perceptions of the fax machine as "archaic," as a "dinosaur technology" (Scott 2019); calls to replace it often point to the demonstrable need for more secure, encrypted, end-to-end communication technologies (Jones 2019; Castillo 2018). They also note the fallibility of faxes, which are prone to various transmission issues that can prove quite serious given the nature of the information that is being communicated. For example, blurring and other degradations in reproductive quality are known issues when it comes to faxed prescriptions (Kelly and Vaida 2004; Feldman et al. 2012). Misdirection is another common transmission problem. In 2019, it came to light that a Melbourne medical clinic had been incorrectly faxing sensitive patient information to a Melbourne man, who inexplicably waited two years before reporting the error (Cunningham 2019). And, in a 2018 Victorian coronial enquiry, it was found that a patient's scans, containing information vital to his cancer treatment, were sent to the wrong fax number (Cunningham 2019). In handing down her findings, Coroner Rosemary Carlin was critical of the continued use of faxes within the Victorian medical profession:

> It is difficult to understand why such an antiquated and unreliable means of communication persists at all in the medical profession. . . . [I]t seems to me that it should be phased out as a means of communicating test results as a matter of priority. (Carlin 2018, 33 § 123)

And, yet, still the fax persists in the Australian healthcare system, as it does in other medical systems (Johnson 2020; Farr 2018) and across other fields (Koehn 2019). One of our research participants, a government agency employee (interviewed in 2019), noted that, in previous research of their own, they counted 145 separate fax machines in a single Victorian hospital. It persists in the Australian medical context despite concerted work by Australian government agencies and various affiliated medical bodies to promote alternative, more "secure" forms of end-to-end encrypted communication. As a medical specialist (interviewed in 2019), pointed out: "[T]he hospitals, they survive on faxes, basically. . . . It's just this big internal fax system."

In this chapter, we draw from a qualitative interview-based study to explore why it is that faxes have come to form such a persistent communication medium within the health care system in Victoria, Australia. Prior to examining reasons for the persistence of fax, it is valuable to first glance back at the history and significance of the fax as a communication and transmission tool.

FAX MACHINES, AND THE TRANSMISSION OF MEDICAL INFORMATION

Development of the fax machine dates to the mid-nineteenth century, with the first patent issued in London in 1843 (Coopersmith 2015, 9). Over successive decades, and right up until the second half of the twentieth century, entrepreneurs and inventors competed in the development and promotion of fax technologies in multiple markets, largely without success (9). It wasn't until the 1980s (following the development of the G3 standard in 1980) that fax really took off and was able to "finally exceed its promoters' promises"

(2). A traditional fax machine works when a sender feeds into the machine a prepared paper document that is then scanned and converted into electrical impulses and transmitted. In the receiving machine, transmitted data is reconverted to impulses and reproduced on paper for the recipient (10). By the mid-1980s, faxing "helped change expectations of information—increasingly including images—from rare to abundant, from hard to find to easy to acquire, from difficult to obtain to simple to create and disseminate" (145–146). The low cost of thermal printing and simple connection via a phone line made the fax machine an office (and home office) staple. Importantly, the fax machine and faxing also dramatically transformed workplaces and work, accelerating "the work cycle from weeks or days to hours or minutes" (161). The 1990s saw the replacement of thermal with plain paper, a shift driven by "the desire for a permanent record . . . without the hassle of making a copy before the thermal fax paper faded" (210).

Faxes have been understood as a truly transformational communication technology (Coopersmith 2015; Light 2006). At the turn of the twentieth century, the fax presented a valuable alternative to standard telegraphy in that it "offered 100-percent accuracy and the authenticity of the original—a major attraction for telegraphers struggling with illegible handwriting, unfamiliar languages, codes, ciphers, and simple human error" (Coopersmith 2015, 16–17); it also promised "the maintenance of secrecy" (17). The promise of accuracy and secrecy have remained steadfast attractions for supporters of the fax (209).

While medical records transfer by fax was explored as early as 1948 (Light 2006, 365), it wasn't until the late 1980s that fax's potential for the health sector was more fully appreciated. In a 1988 trial at Southwest Texas Methodist Hospital, the hospital pharmacy installed fax machines at three nurses' stations in order to "reduce delays in processing prescriptions" (Coopersmith 2015, 169). During this trial, "turnaround dropped from four to eight hours to one hour," tracking of orders was improved, and, as a result, all 36 nurses' stations were equipped with fax machines (169).

Jonathan Coopersmith (2015) argues that digitalization and automation contributed to the decline (if not complete disappearance) in fax use within offices and other large organizations. "After 2000," Coopersmith (2015) writes, "fax seemed an obsolete technology, increasingly replaced as a technological essential by all-digital communications" (207). However, as Jennifer Light (2006) points out, when one looks across the history of the fax, the difficulty one faces in characterizing the fax machine as an old or outdated medium—a "dinosaur technology" (Scott 2019)—is that this history is in fact unfinished.

TECHNOLOGICAL OBDURACY

In exploring this unfinished history of the fax, we draw from Anique Hommels' (2005, 2008) examinations of technological obduracy. Obduracy refers to stubborn persistence, or a state of being resistant to change (inflexibility). Obduracy, Hommels (2005, 324) suggests, has been and continues to be an important critical concern within STS (e.g., Star 1999), where there has been particular interest is understanding the interaction between obduracy and change in sociotechnical developments (Hommels 2005, 330), with the two going hand in hand.

Hommels (2005) draws from the STS literature to develop her own rich account of obduracy, where she develops several important insights that can be summarized as follows.

First, she notes that a useful point of entry in studying technological obduracy and change is to analyze "the role of artifacts as exemplars" of obduracy (2005, 331). We take "artifact" here to mean a technology (or technological assemblage), like the fax.

Second, artifacts are influenced by socially constructed "frames," or ways of thinking about particular technologies (330–331). Frames can play a "constraining role" for specific groups of actors (334), such that "when certain ways of thinking have been built up around an artifact, it becomes difficult to ignore them" (334). Implicit here is "the assumption that because certain ways of thinking have a narrow focus or are difficult to adapt, the technology involved will become obdurate or only have a limited flexibility" (334). And for those heavily invested in a particular technological frame, they think and interact "very much in terms of that technological frame" (331), and it can become difficult to think of alternatives. Hommels describes this as "'closed-in' obduracy" (331). Hommels' core point here is that it is "important to analyze for whom a technological artifact is obdurate and for whom it is not" (331).

Third, the extent to which a particular technological artifact has become *embedded* in infrastructural and other sociotechnical systems "determines its resistance to efforts aimed at changing it" (334). Some technologies are more embedded, and therefore more obdurate and resistant to change, than others. As a rule of thumb, the more embedded technologies become, the greater the difficulty in "changing elements of sociotechnical ensembles" (337). To change one element carries "consequences for (at least a part) of the whole ensemble" (334). This is because "obduracy is no intrinsic property of technologies but can only be understood in the context of its ties to other elements within a network" (334). In short, sociotechnical change is relational.

Fourth, it is also important to look beyond technological frames to wider "contextual" or structural factors that [may] play a role in the construction of obduracy (338), such as larger technological step-changes, or the implications and impacts of regulatory regimes and policy shifts and interventions.

Hommels' interest in obduracy is in regard to urban sociotechnical developments (in particular, see Hommels 2008). Nevertheless, her treatment of obduracy has wider application and is productive for considering what Don Ihde (2019) calls "medical technics," with "technics" understood as "technologies in use and the materiality of technologies" (2019, 2). We see this dual understanding of technics at play in Hommels' analysis of obduracy as thoroughly sociotechnical, including in the sense that technologies can obdure (persist), and in the sense that users of technologies can also be obdurate (intractable, unwilling to change). Sometimes the former is a result of the latter; more commonly, there are a multitude of factors at play, as we explore below.

APPROACH

In this chapter, we ask why it is that faxes persist in hospitals and other health care contexts within the Australian state of Victoria. In responding to this question, we draw on an exploratory study involving ten semi-structured interviews (Green and Thorogood, 2018) conducted over a period of almost ten years, from 2014 to 2023.[1] This extended time period resulted from this unfunded study having to fit around other, larger-scale, funded research projects and other commitments. These interviews with health communication technology consultants, and with health professionals—namely, medical specialists, and allied health professionals (a broad category that includes social workers, physiotherapists, psychologists, among many other roles and professions [Turnbull et al. 2009, 29]). Ten participants might be regarded as a small sample size, yet as Crouch and McKenzie (2006, 483) explain, "since such a project scrutinizes the dynamic qualities of a situation . . . the issue of sample size—as well as representativeness—has little bearing on the project's basic logic." The duration of the study serves to demonstrate the persistence of the fax in medical contexts even as more new technologies come on board, something we could not have anticipated in 2014, but have continued to document with each detailed interview. This ultimately proved advantageous insofar as the issue of fax's presence within the health system in Victoria did not recede nor go away over this period, despite repeated suggestions that it would. To account for this temporal landscape, the year in which interviews were conducted is given when described or quoted from in the chapter.

We initially began interviews by asking healthcare practitioners about their practices of fax machine use and non-use, enquiring into the materiality of the machine, the data cultures around it and the frame of thinking held by the individual and organization, asking questions such as: what do you use the fax for, why do you think that you/your workplace still uses a fax machine, how important would you say faxes are to your work/in your workplace, and why do you think the use of fax machines persists in medical/healthcare contexts? When interviewing health practitioners using fax machines in their daily roles, we invited them to physically demonstrate the use of the machine and talk through the materiality of the device and its situatedness in the workplace. As the project evolved, we interviewed health communication technology consultants and policy makers who spoke to the systemic complexities of fax machine persistence in healthcare contexts.

Practitioners were recruited in Melbourne, where both researchers are based, and were interviewed at their place of work and near their facsimile machine. All were healthcare professionals. Five were in clinical settings, four were medical technology experts, and one was in healthcare system administration. Consultants and policy makers were interviewed at a place of mutual convenience (e.g., a café) or online (via Microsoft Teams). Interviews lasted between 30 and 90 minutes. All participants were recruited according to convenience and snowball sampling (Battaglia 2011) through social media, personal, and professional networks. The methods of recruitment mean that the extent to which our findings can be generalized is limited to this context.

Participants were recruited across public and private healthcare sectors. The Australian healthcare system is a publicly funded system that provides universal access to medical services and hospital care. It is primarily funded by the federal government, as well as state and territory governments, and is managed by the Department of Health. Facsimile machines are part of ensemble of medical technologies employed in the Australian healthcare system that range from paper records to high-end diagnostic equipment, and sit alongside email, secure messaging systems, encrypted medical practice software, photocopiers, fixed-line and mobile phones, and pagers. The focus of interviews was on fax use, specifically, within that ensemble.

INFRASTRUCTURAL EMBEDDEDNESS

In developing this interview-based study, we sought to understand the persistence of the fax and examine impediments to the take-up of modern, encrypted health communications systems. What emerges from the study is a complicated socio-technical picture, with several significant interconnecting issues contributing to the continued presence and ongoing embrace of fax machines and their infrastructural embeddedness and obduracy. We characterize these as *complexities of everyday data cultures*, *technological complexities*, and *systemic complexities*. Each will be examined in turn.

COMPLEXITIES OF EVERYDAY DATA CULTURES

In the UK, the directive to "axe the fax" has proven difficult to implement. Despite bans on the purchase of new faxes, and threats of punitive measures for those who do not comply, removal of faxes was complicated by the fact that they have come to form "an essential network across the NHS—and other healthcare institutions—over decades" (Johnson 2020). The fax had come to constitute a vital connecting technology within a larger health communications ecosystem. This is also the case in Australia, especially Victoria, which has multiple independent healthcare systems. In order to understand why this is the case, it is valuable to consider "technologies as social practice" (Suchman et al. 1999, 392), or what is elsewhere referred to as "everyday data cultures" (Burgess et al. 2022)—how data, and the technologies that collect and transmit data, are "encountered, experienced, exploited and resisted in the practice of everyday life" (4).

Greenhalgh et al. (2019) make two pertinent observations about health information infrastructure. One is that it is "collectively learned, known, and practiced" (3). The other is that, through this, it becomes "embedded" within established organizational systems and ways of doing things. Across all the interviews we conducted with health professionals, fax remained a core communication (and payment-related) technology and was entrenched within daily practice. One of our first interviews was with a payroll manager in a hospital. He explained how the fax machine was essential in the processing of transactions:

> If someone's got a medical certificate that they need to provide pay office so that we can make a payment, they would then send us a fax of their medical certificate. Now we need originals anyway, but in the process of getting things done, we'll organize the payment on a fax, and then chase up the original. (Hospital payroll manager, interviewed in 2014)

Practitioners working in allied services relied on fax to coordinate approval processes between services:

> So, doctors will make an EPC [enhanced primary care] form, which is like a Medicare approval; so, they'll fax it here, and then one of the doctors will have

> to sign it and agree, and then we'll fax it back. (Administrator in an osteopathic clinic, interviewed in 2015)

In this same context, fax was also used a means of processing payment authorization:

> Generally, for TENS [transcutaneous electrical nerve stimulation] machines, they're an electro-based machine . . . we don't actually process the payments here. They [clients] just fill out a form that we fax off to TENS, then they [TENS] process all the payments and it all goes through them. . . . Fax is their preferred means of distributing their product. (Receptionist in a physiotherapy clinic, interviewed in 2015)

In this instance, the fax served as an intermediary, verifying connection between patient, clinic, and specialist equipment supplier.

Use of fax within everyday communication in these contexts was not an anomaly or an exception. Rather, fax use was a regular occurrence, as this specialist described:

> Well, it's the primary communication between GPs and specialists and us [another form of specialist]. So, GPs fax us referrals and we send letters out by fax. . . . There is probably about 100 [faxes being sent each week]. Because often our letters, too, are sent to multiple people, so people who are seeing five specialists, we send letters to five specialists. So, yeah, it's primary communication between GPs and us, and it is also a good [form of] communication for [relaying] urgent results. (Medical specialist, interviewed in 2019)

The experiences of these participants, spanning the Victorian health care sector (from hospitals to allied health), reveal the embeddedness of fax within daily practice. This medical specialist also details how they use specific methods of faxing for different medical processes and services:

> Letters [of referral, etc.] get electronically faxed because they go straight from Genie [a medical practice management software system]. But things like radiology requests, they don't get electronically done. I have to physically do that. . . . If I'm ordering infusions for people, I have to fax it off to the provider, and if I am writing orders for district nursing, so RDNS [Royal District Nursing Service], we fax [instructions] to them all the time. So, you know, "Please give 20 hits of insulin to this patient every morning." That is to get signed and faxed off. So, [fax is] still the primary way that different health care providers communicate, again because of the confidentiality issue and because it is instant and much cheaper than snail mail. (Medical specialist, interviewed in 2019)

These participant observations all reveal the well-embedded, relational (Star and Ruhleder, 1996) character of fax within the Victorian health care system. Within this system, fax has come to constitute a tried-and-tested and relied upon referral and records transfer system, most especially for allied health professionals. It is a technology that has become firmly embedded within the everyday data cultures and health communication practices of hospital workers, specialists, GP clinic staff (especially receptionists), and allied health workers.

The implications of this embeddedness are important for understanding attempts at socio-technical change. The embeddedness reveals that health communication infrastructures can only be understood in relational terms and changing one element of an infrastructural mix impacts "the whole ensemble" (Hommels 2005, 334) in significant ways. Furthermore, the more embedded technologies become, the greater the difficulty in "changing elements of sociotechnical ensembles" (337). Strong investment in an embedded technology can lead to a hardening of attitudes towards change—what's known as "'closed-in' obduracy" (331). We see this, for example, in the following response from an allied health specialist who was very resistant to calls to remove faxes:

> That is one thing that makes me cross: when I hear people who are outside the medical set saying, "oh, it's old-fashioned, it's antiquated. Everybody should get with it." . . . [I]t's annoying when people go, "oh, nobody uses fax anymore." Well, the fact is the medical profession use it extensively, as I believe the legal profession still prefer fax for security reasons. So, that's frustrating when they come up with that sort of comment. (Occupational therapist in private practice, interviewed in 2019)

Obduracy—in this case understood in the sense of worker resistance to change—can also occur at the point at which new technological solutions are introduced, particularly when the initial engagement with the system presents the user with a greater the level of complexity than what the technology is intended to supersede. A clear example of this, relayed to us by a GP with a keen interest in health informatics policy, involved a CEO at a regional hospital investigating why staff within a central triage point had not adopted the new secure messaging system they had been instructed to use, and discovering the following:

> Apparently, the triage administration people had made a unilateral decision that they weren't going to deal with this system because it was too complicated, and that they had then two systems in place at the same time. They just wanted to go to the fax, and that was all they wanted to deal with, and so [the new secure

> messaging system] just gradually faded away. (GP and Practice Technology Management Expert Committee member, interviewed in 2021)

Suchman and colleagues (1999, 399) have noted that "individual technologies add value only to the extent that they are assembled together into effective configurations." For these hospital workers, the new secure messaging system brought additional complication to their established work practices; it did not come to form a constitutive part of an effective configuration that would displace their preference for and familiarity with fax.

TECHNOLOGICAL COMPLEXITIES

A further reason that fax use persists in the Australian healthcare sector is due to "the complexity around secure messaging" (Practice Technology Management Expert Committee member, interviewed in 2021). Secure medical messaging systems have proven difficult to develop and implement (Program Director for a national health agency, interviewed in 2021). Among the many technical difficulties to overcome include establishing *interoperability standards* (getting different systems to talk to each other), *payload standards* (being able to send and receive messages, or information packets, with diverse forms of content), *addressing* (ensuring a message is going to the right recipient), and *receipting* (acknowledging successful arrival of a message) (Program Director, interviewed in 2021).

Medical systems interoperability remains an international health care challenge (KLAS 2023). In the Australian market, there are four main competing secure messaging vendors (Argus, Global Health, HealthLink, and Medical Objects) and around 300 or so different clinical systems used for the generation of medical messaging content. With the four messaging vendors, the challenge has been to get their proprietary systems to interoperate, despite commercial disincentives to do so.

With respect to message content, the challenge has been twofold. First, to develop the means for medical messaging systems to carry different data packet (payload) types beyond just email-like messages, including "pathology results, discharge summaries, specialist letter[s], referrals, orders" (Program Director, 2021), and so on, especially when each clinical system generates these in slightly different formats. Second, to enable these systems, and the data they carry, to interface with and be usable within the clinical systems used by doctors and other health practitioners (Practice Technology Management Expert Committee member, interviewed in 2021). Both challenges reinforce the point that "all data are first shaped by formats" (Koopman et al. 2021, 784).

With addressability, the ambition has been to create a centralized address-book system where addresses for message senders and recipients are not siloed and locked within individual proprietary messaging vendor databases, with the aim that a user of Argus, for example, is able to find the address of someone using HealthLink, and vice versa. With receipting, the drive has been to encourage the industry to implement an acknowledgment system, whereby the sender is notified if/when a message had been sent and received (or not).

At a federal level, the Australian Digital Health Agency has been working for several years to address each of these issues, using a combination of working parties and other forms of collaboration to arrive at stakeholder consensus, alongside targeted use of industry incentives. The result of this work is broad agreement on interoperability standards and payload standards (these standards are encouraged but not mandated or enforced), and resolution of the centralized address book and receipt generation issues.

Even though these technical barriers to secure medical messaging have largely been overcome, this has not (yet) meant the rapid decline or displacement of the fax. When asked why this is the case, a program management specialist (interviewed in 2021) remarked that, to replace fax, the solution has to be better than what's offered; it has to be "easier, quicker, cheaper, more efficient," and at present it is not. In contrast to secure messaging systems, fax remains easy to use and involves low investment (a machine and a phone line). What is more, with the exception perhaps of addressing, fax encounters none of the issues that dogged secure messaging: faxes are payload agnostic (they transmit anything that can be scanned), easily interoperate, and include sent/received acknowledgments. They also continue to be *perceived* by many health practitioners as a more secure option than other alternatives (such as email) regardless of the reality. As one health IT expert told us, email is secure at the receipt end, fax is secure at the transmission end.

A further reason for fax's persistence and obduracy despite these technological advancements has to do with major structural inequalities across the Victorian healthcare sector, with some parts of the sector much better equipped and prepared technologically than others. The Victorian Department of Health has developed a "digital health maturity model" to measure this, with those that are well-advanced in their integration of electronic medical records solutions (for argument's sake, a hospital) regarded has having a higher level of "digital health maturity" than those less-well advanced (such as allied health practitioners). As a program director for a national health agency observes, within allied health, "you've got a myriad of clinical systems," many of which are still "paper-based." Part of the "lift" towards increasing rates of digital health maturity, according to this program director (interviewed in 2021), will be around improving basic digital adoption within the allied health sector. This is a process that is ongoing. However, for the near future at least, fax remains a vital communication medium for allied health practitioners.

SYSTEMIC COMPLEXITIES

It has become something of a truism within infrastructural studies to say that infrastructure is only noticeable when it breaks down (e.g., Horst 2013, 148). In such situations, the hitherto invisible becomes visible again. This conception of infrastructure doesn't always hold for all infrastructure, however, especially health-related infrastructure. As Greenhalgh et al. (2019, 2) observe, health information infrastructure "has a reputation for being convoluted, conservative, failure-prone, and lacking integration, for numerous interacting reasons" (see also Howe et al. 2016). One reason is chronic underfunding of the health sector in Australia, and elsewhere (Hinchliffe, Ore, and Rose 2022; Zhang, Budhdeo, and Ashrafian 2022). Another concerns the systemic complexities associated with particular jurisdictions.

In Australia, the health system is jointly run by all three levels of government: federal, state and territory, and local (Australian Government 2019). Among the key responsibilities of state and territory governments is managing and administering public hospitals (Australian Government 2019). As a result of this, each state and territory has taken its own approach to addressing health communication infrastructure needs. Victoria, for instance, has not mandated a single, encrypted, state-wide health communication system, as other states have done. As one participant, a general practice doctor, who also sits on various medical practice-related technical committees, explains:

> In Queensland, they're digitally connected across the whole state. They use one record system for an individual. It doesn't matter whether you attend Cairns Hospital [in Far North Queensland] or Redcliffe Hospital [1,600 km south of Cairns, just north of Brisbane in South East Queensland]. They can access the same record. Whereas, we can't do that in Victoria. We've got paper records and electronic records and different systems. (GP and Practice Technology Management Expert Committee member, interviewed in 2021)

In contrast to Queensland (and elsewhere), Victoria has many different, disconnected public health systems:

> You've got Austin Health, you've got Western Health, and that's metropolitan. Then you expand it out and you've got [others in regional areas]. There's 60 of those, and they all can do their own thing in Victoria. They're completely independent, and they can't share information at all at present. If you

> get transferred from Ballarat Hospital [115 km northwest of Melbourne] to the Royal Melbourne Hospital, they have to photocopy your paper record and put it in a folder and send it with you down there. They can't transfer digital images of patients' X-rays, blood tests, and so on—it all gets printed out. It's just absurd. (Practice Technology Management Expert Committee member, interviewed in 2021)

For this GP, the severely fractured nature of the Victorian health system reflects a state level "lack of direction." This fracturing is also a legacy of an unsuccessful earlier attempt to implement a state-wide system (Health*SMART*), which the Victorian Auditor-General's Office concluded failed due to "poor planning and inadequate understanding of the complex requirements for designing and implementing clinical ICT systems" (Victorian Auditor-General 2017, 2).

One result of the fragmented and disconnected Victorian public health system is that it has fed an ongoing reliance on the fax as a relatively straightforward and expedient way of transmitting information—of "shuffling paper around" (GP and Practice Technology Management Expert Committee member, interviewed in 2021)—that might otherwise have occurred via a secure records transmission system, were such a system implemented. With no universal arrangement for electronic medical records transfer across diverse health services, there has long been a belief that "faxes worked for hospitals and they were reliable" (Program Director, interviewed in 2021).

Another study participant, a health communication infrastructure consultant interviewed in 2019, also pointed out that there are commercial incentives to be found in, and ecosystem dependencies that would benefit from, maintaining the present, fragmented structure. For instance, he described how Victoria's health services (Eastern Health, Northern Health, etc.) operate as umbrella structures that manage a range of other, smaller health providers, with each of these larger entities competing. For this reason, each umbrella organization wants their own systems to work; they don't necessarily want to share information with other systems. What is more, one Victorian health service might an get "off-the-shelf" IT solution and create their own "instance" of it that does not share data with a second health service system, because the second health service created their own "instance," using the same software, but these two "instances" don't speak to each other.

Then there are satellite organizations and actors. Digital health solutions vendors, for example, benefit from the complexities that come with a complicated health communication ecosystem, and "it is a disincentive for [these] commercial organizations to have [health services] working together and sharing information and sharing knowledge" (health communication infrastructure consultant, interviewed in 2019). As the healthcare communication infrastructure consultant further elaborates, if systems unification occurs,

> even the commercial aspects of healthcare then get impacted, because you might have fewer blood tests, or fewer MRIs, or fewer X-rays. So, the organizations that are actually legitimately profiting from repeat processes also are not interested in consolidation and sharing of information for things like unique patient identifiers. (Health communication infrastructure consultant, interviewed in 2019)

What these participant insights reveal is a complicated multi-stakeholder investment in maintaining the status quo.

In addition to the above, while hospitals sometimes have a reputation for embracing cutting-edge technologies, particularly in the area of diagnostics (think MRI and CT scanners), in other respects they remain technologically quite conservative institutions, not just for their continued use of fax. For instance, one GP revealed that, within certain Victorian hospital outpatients' departments, patient discharge summaries are still being dictated by a doctor, with the dictation then sent to a typing pool where it is typed up and sent back to the doctor to vet, thus delaying the dispatching of patient discharge summaries to general practice clinics by weeks if not months. Thus, according to this participant, "it's not just faxes and emails, it's the in-house systems that are antiquated" and need to be looked at (GP, interviewed in 2021).

In the Victorian medical context, then, technological obduracy—especially around the continued reliance on the fax machine—can be at least partially understood by, and situated within, the systemic complexities that attend and shape the governance of healthcare services at a state level.

CONCLUSION

In this chapter we have drawn from an interview-based study, conducted over a significant timespan, where we spoke to health communication technology consultants and health professionals about the persistence of fax within the Victorian health care context. The portrait that emerged from this study is of a complicated socio-technical picture, with manifold, interconnecting framing issues (at different scales) contributing to the continued presence and ongoing embrace of fax machines. The fax persists due to *complexities of everyday data cultures*, where fax in Victoria (as in the UK) has, over years of use, come to constitute a crucial technology and form of health communication technology infrastructure that is well-embedded across the whole healthcare sector. And, the fax persists due to *technological complexities*, as there is a plethora of proprietary, competing encrypted systems on the market that have long had difficulty speaking to each other. Even though many of the technical difficulties holding back secure messaging have since been addressed, these systems are yet to fully displace fax. A key factor in this is disparities in technology take-up across the whole sector. It also persists in the Victorian healthcare system due to *systemic complexities*, where there are clear industry incentives to maintain the status quo. Victoria has a patchwork of separate health providers, each with their own communications, IT and records systems that don't interoperate, meaning that the fax continues to serve an important function as an internal and external communication and records transferal system.

The social relations, institutions, and beliefs around what constitutes normal and trusted ("encrypted") means of communication between health professionals shape attitudes towards the introduction of newer technologies that appear to "disrupt" these existing arrangements and norms. We sought to draw out this point by examining the continued importance of fax machines to allied health professionals. In talking with allied health professionals, two things became clear. First, the fax remains a vital means of staying in contact with and receiving referrals from more mainstream health providers, such as general practice doctors (GPs). Second, "everyday practices" and "the desires, uncertainties and anxieties that attend these" reveals a great deal about the "scrappiness of our lived data experiences, . . . our engagements with the textures and traces of everyday data" (Burgess et al. 2022, 43), and how these relational engagements shape attitudes to existing technologies and the introduction of new technologies.

We argue that any serious attempt to phase out faxes must account for and accommodate the relational capacities and systems of networks that are built around and rely upon these established technologies. The technological artifact's embeddedness in infrastructural and other sociotechnical systems "determines its resistance to efforts aimed at changing it" (Hommels 2005, 334). As noted early in this chapter, one hospital had 145 separate fax machines in 2019, yet a health IT consultant participant interviewed more recently (in 2023) noted that now, many of these individual machines have now gone (or are going) but these fax numbers remain and are now routed via a centralized fax server. So, things have changed, but not as much as one might expect.

NOTE

1. Interviews for this project were suspended during the height of the COVID-19 pandemic. In 2020 and 2021, Melbourne experienced six lockdown periods, and the

Victorian health system was operating under severe strain. Conducting fieldwork involving medical practitioners was not feasible over this period.

REFERENCES

Australian Government. 2019. The Australian Health System. The Australian Government: Department of Health and Aged Care. https://www.health.gov.au/about-us/the-australian-health-system

Battaglia, M. (2011). "Convenience Sampling." In *Encyclopedia of Survey Research Methods*, edited by Paul J. Lavrakas, 149–150. Thousand Oaks, CA: Sage.

Burgess, Jean, Kath Albury, Anthony McCosker, and Rowan Wilken. 2022. *Everyday Data Cultures*. Cambridge: Polity.

Carlin, Rosemary. 2018. *Finding into Death with Inquest [of Mettaloka Malinda Halwala]* (Ref. no. COR 2015 5857). Coroner's Court of Victoria. https://www.coronerscourt.vic.gov.au/sites/default/files/2018-12/mettalokamalindahalwala_585715.pdf

Castillo, Luis. 2018. "Death of the Fax Machine: Three IT Challenges Standing in the Way of Fax's Ultimate Destruction." *Forbes*, September 17. https://www.forbes.com/sites/forbestechcouncil/2018/09/17/death-of-the-fax-machine-three-it-challenges-standing-in-the-way-of-faxs-ultimate-destruction/?sh=3a7adc16523b

Coopersmith, Jonathan. 2015. *Faxed: The Rise and Fall of the Fax Machine.* Baltimore: Johns Hopkins University Press.

Cunningham, Melissa. 2019. "'Detailed and Graphic': Clinic Faxes Patients' Highly Sensitive Medical Histories to Wrong Number." *The Age*, September 18. https://www.theage.com.au/national/victoria/detailed-and-graphic-clinic-faxes-patients-highly-sensitive-medical-histories-to-wrong-number-20190916-p52rsy.html

digitalhealth.gov.au. 2019. "Axe the Fax: New Agency Incentive Supports Paperless Healthcare." *digitalhealth.gov.au*, March 27. https://www.digitalhealth.gov.au/newsroom/media-releases/archived-media-releases/axe-fax-new-agency-incentive-supports-paperless

Farr, Christina. 2018. "Fax Machines are Still Common in Medicine—and Med Students are Puzzled When Forced to Use This Ancient Technology." *CNBC*, February 10. https://www.cnbc.com/2018/02/10/milllennial-doctors-forced-to-use-fax-machines-causing-puzzlement.html

Feldman, Henry J., Homoud Al-Jalahma, Rashid Al-Ali, and Shane Reti. 2012. "Faxed Arabic Prescriptions: A Medication Error Waiting to Happen?" *International Journal of Medical Informatics* 81, no. 3: 192–195.

Green, Judith M., and Nicki Thorogood. 2018. *Qualitative Methods for Health Research*, 4th ed. London: Sage.

Greenhalgh, Trisha, Joseph Wherton, Sara Shaw, Chrysanthi Papoutsi, Shanti Vijayaraghavan, and Rob Stones. 2019. "Infrastructure Revisited: An Ethnographic Case Study of How Health Information Infrastructure Shapes and Constrains Technological Innovation." *Journal of Medical Internet Research* 21, no. 12: 1–19. https://www.jmir.org/2019/12/e16093/

Hinchliffe, Joe, Adeshola Ore, and Tamsin Rose. 2022. "End of 50–50 Hospital Funding Deal with States to Have 'Devastating' Impact, Australia's Peak Bodies Say." *The Guardian*, October 27. https://www.theguardian.com/australia-news/2022/oct/27/end-of-50-50-hospital-funding-deal-with-states-to-have-devastating-impact-australias-peak-bodies-say

Hommels, Anique. 2005. "Studying Obduracy in the City: Toward a Productive Fusion Between Technology Studies and Urban Studies." *Science, Technology & Human Values* 30, no. 3: 323–351.

Hommels, Anique. 2008. *Unbuilding Cities: Obduracy in Urban Sociotechnical Change*. Cambridge, MA: MIT Press.

Horst, Heather A. 2013. "The Infrastructures of Mobile Media: Towards a Future Research Agenda." *Mobile Media & Communication* 1, no. 1: 147–152.

Howe, Cymene, Jessica Lockrem, Hannah Appel, Edward Hackett, Dominic Boyer, Randal Hall, Matthew Schneider-Mayerson, Albert Pope, Akhil Gupta, Elizabeth Rodwell, Andrea Ballestero, Trevor Durbin, Farès el-Dahdah, Elizabeth Long, and Cyrus Mody. 2016. "Paradoxical Infrastructures: Ruins, Retrofit, and Risk." *Science, Technology, & Human Values* 41, no. 3: 547–565.

Ihde, Don. 2019. *Medical Technics*. Minneapolis, MN: University of Minnesota Press.

Johnson, Matthew. 2020. "Don't 'Axe the Fax.'" *Opentext*, September 30. https://blogs.opentext.com/dont-axe-the-fax/

Jones, Frank. 2019. "Fax Machine, Rest in Peace." *NAB*. https://web.archive.org/web/20210118230608/https://www.nab.com.au/business/industry/healthcare/managing-a-practice/fax-machine-rest-in-peace

Kelly, Kate, and Allen J. Vaida. 2004. "'Fax Noise' Can Result in Medication Errors." *Pharmacy Times*, July 1. https://www.pharmacytimes.com/view/2004-07-8054

Kerr, Richard. 2020. "Axe the Fax: Bringing About the End of the Outdated Hospital Machinery." *National Health Executive*, February 3. https://www.nationalhealthexecutive.com/Health-Service-Focus/axe-the-fax-bringing-about-the-end-of-the-outdated-hospital-machinery

KLAS. 2023. *Interoperability Summit 2022: White Paper*. *KLAS Research*. https://klasresearch.com/report/interoperability-summit-2022/2885

Koehn, Emma. 2019. "The Simple Fax: This 'Dinosaur' of Tech Isn't Dead Yet." *The Age*, January 7. https://www.theage.com.au/business/small-business/the-simple-fax-this-dinosaur-of-tech-isn-t-dead-yet-20181217-p50mn6.html

Koopman, Colin, Patrick Jones, Valérie Simon, Paul Showler, and Mary McLevey. 2021. "When Data Drive Health: An Archaeology of Medical Records Technology." *BioSocieties* 17: 782–804. https://doi.org/10.1057/s41292-021-00249-1

Light, Jennifer S. 2006. "Facsimile: A Forgotten 'New Medium' from the 20th Century." *New Media & Society* 8, no. 3: 355–378.

Scott, Elise. 2019. "Fax Machines are Being Kept on Life Support by Canberra's Health System Despite Calls for Change." *ABC News*, June 23. https://www.abc.net.au/news/2019-06-23/fax-machines-being-kept-on-life-support-by-act-health/11236778

Star, Susan Leigh. 1999. "The Ethnography of Infrastructure." *American Behavioral Scientist* 43, no. 3: 377–391.

Star, Susan Leigh, and Karen Ruhleder. 1996. "Steps Towards an Ecology of Infrastructure: Design and Access for Large Information Spaces." *Information Systems Research* 7, no. 1: 111–134.

Suchman, Lucy, Jeanette Blomburg, Julian E. Orr, and Randall Trigg. 1999. "Reconstructing Technologies as Social Practice." *American Behavioral Scientist* 43, no. 3: 392–408.

Turnbull, Catherine, Karen Grimmer-Somers, Saravana Kumar, Esther May, Deborah Law, and Elaine Ashworth. 2009. "Allied, Scientific and Complementary Health Professionals: A New Model for Australian Allied Health." *Health Professional Education* 33, no. 1: 27–37.

Victorian Auditor-General. 2017. *ICT Strategic Planning in the Health Sector: Victorian Auditor-General's Report*. Victorian Auditor-General's Office, May. Melbourne: Victorian Government Printer.

Zhang, J., S. Budhdeo, and H. Ashrafian. 2022. "Failing IT Infrastructure is Undermining Safe Healthcare in the NHS." *The BMJ*, 379. https://doi.org/10.1136/bmj-2022-073166

PART II

Envisioning the Body through Technology

Chapter 3

The Fetal Scan Project

Anna Gonzalez Suero

This essay is an autoethnographic study of an artistic project I worked on together with pregnant people. The fetal scan project, which took place in 2015, was carried out in the German city of Cologne over a period of three months. This essay reflects on my experiences during those months. For the fetal scan project, I offered to work for pregnant people, to do their housework or other work, following a feminist idea about wages for housework. But instead of receiving a wage in return, I wanted to get their take-home fetal ultrasound image which they are socially expected to cherish as a precious keepsake.

In Germany, as in other countries, ultrasound examinations are routinely performed on pregnant patients to track fetal growth. Besides having a diagnostic value, ultrasound examinations allow pregnant patients to view real-time, moving images of the fetus on a computer screen and to take home with them printouts for personal use. I wanted to get from pregnant people this take-home keepsake fetal image. By then, I had already spent almost fifteen years drawing artistic fetal forms by hand. Many of my artistic fetal forms were made of paper and wood, which are traditional materials. Elsewhere I have written about the artistic creation of a handmade form I call "fetus-phallus" (Gonzalez Suero 2022a). After reworking the phallus as an extension of my larger artistic practice with fetal forms, I now wanted to repurpose the manufactured, technical image of the growing fetus generated by the ultrasound machine. So I decided that I needed to get other people's fetal scans and that, for this to happen, I would take it upon myself to work for them. A series of unusual but necessary exchanges began to unfold in the context of my fetal scan project. These out-of-the-ordinary exchanges, in turn, revealed to me the individual needs of pregnant people.

In what follows, I want to reconstruct from memory how and why I tried to change the social norm of saving the fetal scan as a keepsake. What new meaning, if at all, did the fetal scan acquire within this artistic project? To contextualize my personal story about working with and for the fetal scans of pregnant people as an artist, I will engage with feminist debates on reproductive technologies and imagery, which analyze the techno-scientific construction of the fetus through its visualization and medicalization. I also aim to situate my artistic use of the fetal scan in a historical context and in relation to socioeconomic factors and political issues.

The autoethnographic study presented below is based on memories. To recall my memories, I have worked with the technique which Carolyn Ellis (1991, 2004, 2008) calls "systematic sociological introspection," with the aim of gaining new insights regarding those memories. Ellis (2004, 37) is well-known for developing a widely accepted definition of autoethnography which describes it as "writing about the personal and its relationship to culture." Systematic sociological introspection, which is "the primary method connected with autoethnographic writing," involves a "self-dialogue" or "inner conversation" in which one revisits memories of past experiences (Ellis 2008, 853–854). I wrote down my memories and then used them as raw material to construct an "autoethnographic fiction" (Ellis 2004, 332). There is an inventive aspect to autoethnographic writing since it requires one to select, to edit, and to reshape memories of real events using fictional devices like characterization, plot, dialogue, and metaphor.

And indeed in the process of writing down my personal memories and turning them into an autoethnographic fiction, I have become aware of previously overlooked aspects of the fetal scan project, some of which are discussed below. Doing so has deepened my understanding of how a cultural icon, in this case the ultrasound image of the fetus, can have different meanings depending on the specific social and economic situation of the particular pregnant person who gestates the fetus that is iconized. By showing the diverse contexts of ultrasound images of the fetus, my autoethnographic fiction aims to contribute to feminist scholarship that challenges the presumed autonomy of the fetal icon.

PREGNANT? I WANT YOU!

In 2015, on a March spring day, I rode my bike to the University Hospital of Cologne, one of the largest hospitals in Germany. On the hospital bulletin board I placed my flyer asking pregnant people to participate in my fetal scan project. "Pregnant? I want you!" was the headline for the flyer. I found then several pregnant people. The pregnant person I worked for the most was an

African migrant woman from Ghana who arrived in Germany that year when more than one million migrants arrived. Her name was Maggie.[1]

Maggie is the first person I think about when I look in retrospect at the fetal scan project. Maggie arrived in Cologne when she was eight months pregnant. On the day we met she told me she wanted to participate in my project, the artistic fetal scan project. Maggie, who was in a difficult situation without her own apartment, asked me to find her a two-room apartment. She had a fetal scan and I said yes, I want to work for you.

I began searching for an apartment for Maggie in Cologne, a city with a massive housing shortage. The housing shortage was only getting worse in this year and Maggie was due to give birth to her first child the following month. While we had an agreement, it was unclear whether I could fulfill my part of the agreement.

During the fetal scan project, Maggie was not the only person I worked for. Before I met Maggie, I had already received a phone call from a man named Michael.

"I want you to meet my girlfriend," Michael said quietly to me over the phone. I could barely hear him. I asked him to speak louder and to put his girlfriend on the phone. But he just kept on speaking with a low voice, softly, like he was hiding something. I asked him where he wanted us to meet. "At the hospital where you placed the flyer for your project," he said. "Does your girlfriend want to participate in my project?" I asked him. But Michael did not answer me. Instead, he told me the name of his girlfriend. "I want you to meet Susan."

When I taped my flyer to the wall of the hospital, I had no idea who would give me their fetal scan and what they would want in return. There was written: "I will work for you, do your housework, or something else, in exchange for a print of your fetal scan." The flyer was a paper flyer with tear-off strips with my telephone number.

I came up with the project idea while reading about a small feminist collective that began in the early 1970s in Italy to demand that housework be paid work. This "Wages for Housework" group argued that housework—cleaning, cooking, rearing children, what mostly women have done inside the home, is in fact real work that should be paid (see Federici 1975). To this day housework remains largely undervalued (Weeks 2011). I identified with this second-wave feminist argument not as a "housewife" but as an artist whose profession tends to be romanticized, often stereotypically seen as a vocation or inner calling rather than real work. From this feminist position I composed the content of the flyer for the project. I thought the flyer was good, it was easy to read. On the flyer I also made clear that the project participants had to agree to let themselves be photographed and depicted on a project website.

When I rode my bike to the hospital to meet Michael and his girlfriend Susan, I asked myself again why Michael was acting secretive over the phone. Upon seeing them next to my flyer, I felt reassured and excitedly walked towards them. They smiled. We shook hands.

"I just got off from work," Michael said to me. "I work here in the hospital as a cleaner." "Nice," I said politely and continued, "it seems a nice hospital." We talked some more about this large university hospital, recognized for its ability to provide top-notch care to pregnant patients. I then asked them whether they had received a fetal scan from this hospital or another one.

"Not yet," they responded and hesitated for a moment. "Since getting engaged, we've been trying to become pregnant but can't. We thought you may be able to help."

"Me?" I said. "Why do you think I can help you? You may need to see a doctor."

"No," Michael said. "An artist is better than a doctor."

"Oh, nobody has told me that before," I answered.

Michael looked in my eyes. "You make art and being creative is important." "I'm glad he called you," Susan added. "Michael and I have heard about a powerful aphrodisiac we can't get hold of. It's called maca. We have to take maca. It's that simple. If you find maca for us, we'll give you what you want."

"Well, I don't know where to get maca," I said. "But I might know someone who does."

Lepidium meyenii, commonly known as maca, is an ancient Peruvian plant still consumed today for its fertility-enhancing properties. I knew an artist from Peru, so I called her up and I told her about my meeting with Michael and Susan. By chance, she had a friend who worked here in the city with the maca plant. Over the phone she told me the story of Dolores, a medical student who had been working in the Andes Mountains, digging in the soil to collect the white maca root. Dolores packed her suitcase with as much maca as she could fit. She then carried the heavy suitcase to Cologne, where she had been trying to scientifically prove the sexual benefits of maca. To help pay for her doctoral studies, she was also selling maca on the side. "It's thanks to Dolores that I got pregnant," said my friend whose child was one month old at the time.

A few days later I met Dolores and we travelled with the maca powder to where Michael and Susan lived. Dolores gave them a small plastic bag with the amber-colored maca powder. She sold them a hundred grams for a special price of fifteen euros.

I asked Michael and Susan if I could photograph them posing in their kitchen with the maca power. I wanted to show how they consumed the maca powder with yogurt, trying to become pregnant. They blushed and shook their heads, as though it was something to be ashamed about. With their permission I made two or three photographs of them without the maca powder and then put my camera away. This was the final documentation of my first "housework." But I didn't get a fetal scan for that.

Months later, I heard that Michael and Susan bought more maca powder from Dolores and kept on ordering more and more without becoming pregnant. Their story of ordering more and more maca could be read as one of "hope," or as "hope management," a term proposed by Sarah Franklin in her well-discussed ethnography *Embodied Progress: A Cultural Account of Assisted Conception*, published in 1997. Franklin was one of the first feminist anthropologists to analyze the rise of infertility services in the late 1980s in Britain to treat reproductive health–related problems in individuals who want to have biological children. In her 1997 ethnographic study of British couples' experiences of in-vitro fertilization (IVF), she found that many of them were aware of the low success rate but nevertheless wanted to try it and to try again after it had failed. Franklin identified and analyzed how narratives of hope were mobilized by the infertile couples she interviewed as they underwent repeated IVF treatment without success. To increase the chances of success, female patients are given fertility drugs early on in the IVF process, before their eggs are retrieved from their bodies. The IVF process involves fertilizing an egg with a sperm in a glass dish in a laboratory, then transferring the embryo back into the female body. Reflecting on the exhausting nature of the treatment process, Franklin (1997, 158–159) developed the term "hope management." This term, following Franklin, points to how her interviewees' strong belief in technological progress and scientific knowledge motivated them to go through the IVF process in the first place and to keep on going and having faith in it even when it did not work for them.

Since the publication of Franklin's 1997 study on assisted reproductive technology, interest and demand for the technology has dramatically grown in many parts of the world, with the effect that technology is now widely seen as part of the "natural" process of biological reproduction (Knecht, Klotz, and Beck 2012). Maca, which has been consumed by Andean people for centuries, began to gain popularity beyond Peru in the late 1990s, following and possibly in response to the emergence of assisted reproductive technologies (Gonzales 2011). Promoted on the global market as a "natural" alternative remedy to clinical treatment, which requires taking synthetic hormones, maca has risen to prominence despite only a few scientific studies proving its efficacy (Beharry and Heinrich 2018). Maca, I argue, is perhaps as much a "hope technology" as IVF (Franklin 1997, 192).

After my first "housework" for Michael and Susan, I waited for more people to react to my flyer and eventually I got a call from a social worker who saw my flyer at the hospital and ripped off a paper strip. On the phone the social worker said to me: "Some of the African migrant women I work for are pregnant, yet most are superstitious when it comes to pregnancy. They believe that pregnant women are easily susceptible to evil spirits and therefore tend to avoid contact with strangers. But we could try to convince them to participate in your fetal scan project during the next group meeting that will take place on Friday. They are in need of help."

During the African migrant group meeting on the following Friday, I described what a fetal scan is. "A fetal scan is a normative and technical image produced by high-frequency sound waves." I stood in front of the group, showed them pictures of ultrasound machines and added, "A vast amount of feminist research has been carried out on how parents are socially expected to hold on to a print of their fetal scan as a way of bonding with the fetus at home. An important essay, which is widely cited as marking the beginning of feminist research into prenatal technology, is Rosalind Pollack Petchesky's 'Fetal Images: The Power of Visual Culture.' When 'Fetal Images' was published in 1987, almost thirty years ago, expectant parents were just starting to develop a social identity for their fetus through sharing their fetal scans with a broader public, producing what Petchesky termed a 'public fetus.' Today, there are many pregnant people posting their fetal scans online. This social practice, seen from a feminist perspective, normalizes the idea that fetuses are individuals."

Then I tried to explain to the group why I was interested in their fetal scans. I said: "As an artist I want to open a creative space for pregnant people to experience their fetal scans in less individualistic ways that are not normative or conformist. Feminist and other pro-choice advocates are urgently calling for artists to help debunk the illusion of fetal autonomy through the creation of new visual images that show the dependency of the fetus on the pregnant person. I have already worked for many years with the iconic form of the fetus, creating artistic variations of this form in drawings, photographs, collages, and videos. My last project interrogated the iconic fetal form by visually attaching it to the phallic image of the penis, and in my new art project, the fetal scan project, I want to bring the lived experiences of the pregnant individual into focus."

I took a short breath, then I explained my idea in more detail. "I will document in photographs the housework I do for you. These photographs will then be posted on a project website[2] and contextualized with key feminist writings on fetal scans. For example, I will make reference to Petchesky's 1987 essay, which I discussed before."

I paused to look around the room at their faces. The woman next to me was staring at my fingernails, which I had grown impressively long with very pointy tips. I wasn't sure about cutting my fingernails and now I realized I should have. I was nervous and I knew I was trying too hard to convince them that my intentions were good.

After collecting my thoughts I continued to talk about how their fetal scans could serve many other purposes depending on what they needed most right now. But then the woman next to me suggested that I would do voodoo with their fetal scans. At this point, the social worker got angry and raised her voice: "It's only a picture, a technical picture." "Yes," I said, "it's only a picture."

I WANT A TWO-BEDROOM APARTMENT

At the African migrant group meeting, I met Maggie. When everyone else had gone home, Maggie told me that what kept the other pregnant women in the group from taking part in the project was the belief that I could be a "witch."

A few days later I showed an article to Maggie about witch camps for African women accused of inducing sexual and economic sterility. After Maggie told me she didn't believe in witches, I came across this article online about the return of witch-hunting in the northern part of Ghana, where Maggie came from. I asked her about the witch camps, but she never heard of them. We rode the bus to our first apartment viewing and I showed her the article on my phone display. She shook her head and said, "I don't know anything about it." The article, titled "Witch-Hunting, Globalization, and Feminist Solidarity in Africa Today," was written in 2008 by the Italian feminist scholar, teacher, and activist Silvia Federici, who was amongst the founders of the "Wages for Housework" campaign in the early 1970s.

Before Maggie left Ghana, she was able to claim European citizenship by descent. Many years ago, when I was Maggie's age, I too obtained European citizenship through ancestry from Spain. But Maggie's boyfriend, Sam, didn't have that possibility. He had to cross the Mediterranean Sea to Italy, travelling what has been widely reported to be one of the deadliest routes to Europe.

Sam was with us on our first apartment viewing. They wanted to move into an apartment together. There in the apartment, Maggie and Sam walked in and out, back and forth, room to room. They said they wanted to move into the apartment immediately. I asked them again where they were currently staying. But they didn't want to tell me. All they said was that they didn't like the people they were living with.

We stood in a line with other applicants who were also eager to get the apartment and were waiting to speak to the landlord. While waiting Sam told me that he had been trying to learn German. Maggie said that the constant worry about the apartment made it hard for her to concentrate on learning a new language. After a short wait the landlord said, "It's a tricky process, you still need to locate some more documents, and there are many other people interested, as you can see."

It took us a whole day to collect the required documents from the town hall. In the days that followed we visited more apartments. Most were in bad condition. And Maggie, who was living on unemployment benefits, couldn't afford a better one. It was a hot day, and Maggie had difficulty walking in the heat. We didn't find an apartment during these days. And so, I continued to search the internet for rentals, to view pictures of apartments online, to make phone calls to landlords, and to set up as many appointments as possible.

Then on another hot day we visited an apartment that didn't look anything like the images on the internet. "We're wasting time on ugly apartments," said Maggie, adding that the apartment we just saw had only one and a half bedrooms, not two. "Are you sure the apartment we're heading for will be nice?" I didn't answer her. I thought as she spoke there was doubt in her voice. She seemed not to understand how high the competition for apartments was, even for people who have lived here for a long time. Walking around in this heat wave, I tried to be patient and understanding, but Maggie was now again questioning my competence. She went on, "Do you know where we are now?"

I glanced at the map on my phone, trying to navigate around this neighborhood I'd never been before. My battery was running low. And it was true, I wasn't a good navigator with maps. The map app showed me that we were still twenty minutes away. "C'mon, it's not far away," I said and tried to reassure Maggie that we were not lost. "I know the way; we'll be there soon."

Eventually, we reached the apartment which was for rent. "This is it," I said and smiled at Maggie. She looked stressed. I rang the doorbell and at the sound of the buzzer, I pushed the door open and held it open for Maggie. With my phone I filmed how Maggie entered the concrete building block and how she walked up the floors of the building. I stayed behind her to film how she reached the fourth floor and how she shouted from upstairs, "We don't have time to waste."

We didn't get that apartment either. We had more hard days ahead of us and at some point during our tough time together I really didn't think I could find an apartment for her. To try to deal with this uneasy feeling, I started to work during my free time on the project website. By now I had taken many photographs of Maggie. Sitting at my desk at night I posted a picture and then I really got into it and posted another and continued posting more to create a visual story of our time together.

"We have to tell your story through visuals," I told Maggie on one of those days. "We need to produce more content for the project website," I said on another day as we hurried through the city to the social welfare office. We were hurrying because we were late for the appointment. "We need to ask them for more money, we can't be late," Maggie answered me as she picked up her pace. I took a picture of us running across the street as the light was turning red.

After a long day I arrived late at home. While picking up my room I thought about what Maggie said to me earlier that day. She said she decided to leave her home in Ghana when she was one month pregnant. "I left my home because the public health system there is bad and only wealthy people can afford a good hospital," she said. "But in Germany the public health system takes care of you. It's my right to receive the best-possible prenatal care." The German healthcare system, I thought, might take care of her, but she still needs a place to live here in this city.

In retrospect I think that Maggie wanted to have the chance to give birth in a sophisticated clinic with superior technical equipment, hoping this would ensure the birth of a "healthy" and "normal" child. Her story about moving from Ghana to Germany to optimize her pregnancy outcome could be seen as an example of the way that socially constructed categories of race and class shape an individual's experience of pregnancy and birth. Maggie seemed to feel more socially included through receiving medical benefits in Germany which were otherwise inaccessible to her in Ghana. Her relationship to prenatal technology and to the medicalization of her pregnancy was, in retrospect, similar to that of the interviewed pregnant people in the ethnographic study *Reproducing Race: An Ethnography of Pregnancy as a Site of Racialization*, carried out by feminist law professor Khiara Bridges in 2011.

In *Reproducing Race* (2011), Bridges offers some insights into the role of race and class for low-income pregnant people of color dependent on Medicaid, a social welfare program in the United States. Her study utilizes participant observation and interviews to analyze the situation of uninsured pregnant people receiving government assistance for their prenatal care at Alpha Hospital, the largest public hospital in New York City. The pregnant people she interviewed were temporarily offered the most technologically sophisticated health services. The reason why the federal government expands health insurance coverage to uninsured pregnant people is related to the social construction of the fetus as a person. As Bridges and other feminist scholars have argued, ultrasound technology makes the fetus visually accessible and knowable to obstetricians, and having the fetus as a medical patient gives obstetricians the right to perform many tests on the pregnant individual on the basis that it is "good" for the fetus. While the notion of fetal personhood also affects higher-income individuals, the publicly insured patients at Alpha Hospital, Bridges argues, do not really have the option to choose the model of prenatal care they receive. Bridges makes a comparison between the pregnancies of the privately insured and the publicly insured, arguing that the privately insured can choose between a home birth or the hospital, whereas the publicly insured are not given the option. Following Bridges, the publicly insured must accept the predominant biomedical model of pregnancy or go without prenatal care. It is, to Bridges (2011, 96), a sharp reminder that the pregnancies of people who are of low socioeconomic status are constructed as "always capable of failing," that is, as "unruly bodies."

Bridges, in *Reproducing Race*, describes how, as part of the prenatal care program at Alpha Hospital, the Medicaid-insured patient must be screened for STDs, then tested for gestational diabetes, then undergo an ultrasound scan, then be counseled about how to practice family planning. A "healthy" pregnancy must result, the fetus must be "normal" (Bridges 2011, 156–163). However, as Bridges (2011, 254–257) suggests, their acceptance of the biomedical model of pregnancy can be viewed as an "act of resistance" against social structures that discourage low-income people of color from having "healthy" and "normal" children. Prenatal technology, in Bridges' (2011, 262n1) analysis, serves as a "*technology of inclusion*" when it becomes the medium through which lower-income individuals receive the same medical attention that is usually reserved for wealthier patients. And yet, driving the overmedicalization and hypervisibility of their pregnancies, following Bridges, is structural racism and classism itself. Bridges (2011, 5) concludes that although most of her interviewees benefited from a medically managed pregnancy, the medicalization of their pregnancies gradually took over their lives, making them "both the victims and the beneficiaries" of the public health system.

As in the United States, pregnancy in Germany is constructed as pathological and consequently medicalized (Erikson 2001, 2007, 2015; Samerski 2011, 2015; Sänger 2015). However, feminist scholars call attention to how much more medicalized pregnancy is in Germany, where 70–80 percent of all pregnancies were labeled "at risk" in 2015 (Erikson 2015). Unlike in the United States, where there is no mandate for health insurance at a federal level, all citizens and legal residents in Germany are required by law to have health insurance, regardless of whether they are employed or not employed. Within the German public healthcare system, lower-income individuals have equal access to the same medical services as higher-income individuals, a system which is based on the principle of solidarity.

DECORATING A WINDOW

In the meantime, I received a call from a German woman named Louise. I had just gotten off the phone with a landlord to arrange a date for viewing another apartment for Maggie when Louise called me. On the phone Louise said she tore off a strip of paper from my flyer at the hospital. She was now calling to tell me about the boutique she owns in a trendy district of the city and how she could use my help in getting the store window ready for the upcoming fashion week. "I sell one-of-a-kind garments," Louise continued, "it takes an artist with creative abilities to know how to display these garments in the window. Could you help me with this?" Louise wanted my help to decorate her store window and added that she had many fetal scans she could give me.

After hanging up the phone I wondered why Louise had more than the three standard scans which is considered normal in Germany. I did some research and found a feminist study by Susan Erikson, a medical anthropologist recognized for her research on prenatal technology use in Germany. For her 2001 study, Erikson attended 450 prenatal ultrasound exams as a participant observer in two different German hospitals. Erikson (2001, 210) found that pregnant patients tend to receive extra scans that are not documented in the official *Mutterpass* ("maternity passport"), a handheld record book in which pregnant patients keep their medical data. More recently, in an interview about the current situation of prenatal care in Germany, Erikson (2015) stated that pregnancies previously considered "normal" are without medical reason labeled and treated as being "at risk," subjecting patients to regular monitoring unnecessarily. This is problematic, as it can be a source of anxiety and stress (Erikson 2015).

In another study, "Fetal Views: Histories and Habits of Looking at the Fetus in Germany" (2007), Erikson describes how the act of looking through the pregnant body at the fetus was normalized over time, arguing that it was a gradual process that took place over five centuries, beginning in the sixteenth century when visual representations of the fetus in utero began to appear in midwifery books published across Europe. Prior to this period, the fetus was rarely represented in visual form (see also Sasson and Law 2009). The fetus was an invisible entity, shrouded in secrecy and the unknown. Pregnancy did not exist until there was quickening, a now outdated word that describes the fetal movement as experienced by the pregnant individual (see also Duden 1993). Yet, as midwifery books became popular throughout Europe, visual representations of the fetus began to reach a broader public (see also Whiteley 2023).

Following Erikson (2007) and other feminist scholars, traditional childbirth was a home-based ritual that took place under the care of midwives. The midwifery model of care is very different from contemporary obstetrics, for it defines and treats pregnancy and birth as normal physiological processes. In the early modern period, the general focus of midwifery books was on the moment of birth rather than on the development of the fetus in utero. The role of the midwife was to assist throughout the labor and delivery by touching rather than looking at the pregnant body. It was common belief that birth pains served a natural function (see also Leavitt 1986). A midwife intervened only when there were complications. In these difficult situations, the fetus was understood as being in an unnatural position, that is, in the other-than-head-down position. The fetal representations printed in midwifery books were accompanied by descriptions about how midwives could use their hands to put the fetus back into what was considered a natural position. In such midwifery books, the fetus was understood to be part of the pregnant body and therefore not a separate patient to be looked at.

This reliance on touch began to diminish in the nineteenth century with the development of the modern speculum and other medical technologies. A speculum is a device composed of two hinged blades of concave metal or plastic which looks like a duckbill and is used to open and hold the vaginal walls apart, allowing for visual inspection of the vagina and cervix. Despite its possible health benefits, feminist scholar Margarete Sandelowski, author of "This Most Dangerous Instrument: Property, Power, and the Vaginal Speculum" (2000), has shown that the speculum was made possible only through sexist, racist, and classist practices. Although variations of the speculum trace back to ancient Greece, the American doctor James Marion Sims is widely credited with developing the modern model still in use today. In her 2000 study of the vaginal speculum, Sandelowski, a professor in the School of Nursing at the University of North Carolina at Chapel Hill, describes how Sims fashioned the duck-billed model in the 1840s by using female slaves as test subjects (see also Kapsalis 1997). As Sandelowski (2000: 78) points out, it was not until Sims optimized the speculum on enslaved female subjects that he began to apply it on white, middle- and upper-class female patients.

Before Sims' speculum came into use, it was expected that female patients, including those who were pregnant, would remain clothed while being examined, in accordance with the norms of femininity (see also Prescott 2003). The visual technology of the speculum, Sandelowski argues, contributed to a shift from touching to looking inside the pregnant body. That shift toward a visual mode of knowing is still taking place today, through the ultrasound image of the fetus, with the difference that it requires "viewers to interpret what they do not directly see" (Sandelowski 2000, 79).

After borrowing more feminist books from the library, I rode my bike to meet Louise at her boutique in one of the most fashionable areas of Cologne. On my way there I thought about how being labeled "at risk" transforms pregnant subjects into "housewives" because managing risks is a never-ending task like housework. I spent the day with Louise decorating her store window. While arranging handmade jewelry behind the glass window, Louise described all the details of the ultrasound exam. "The sonographer said my baby was in a perfect position and then he took so many pictures. He was like a paparazzi, taking them as fast as he could. After several scans were printed, I asked him if my fetus was a pop icon."

Late in the evening, when the window display was almost ready for the upcoming fashion week, Louise showed me her collection of fetal scans. They were not the more common and well-known grainy black and white prints. They were of an outstanding quality, colored and in high resolution, showing a crystal clear but partly fragmented fetus. Her fetal scans were printed on glossy photo paper and were the size of a standard photo in a traditional family album. But they were something unfamiliar, some kind of hyperrealistic fetus. Its skin color was not the transparent cloudy grey of the ordinary kind. It was a dense pinkish brown, an artificial color rendered by the software. Its flesh, around the edges of its mouth, had a bumpy texture, rounded like a plastic product, almost like a toy. But certain parts of the clinically pure body of the fetus seemed to be tightly wrapped in rubber. It was a mix of perfect and broken, sometimes with clusters of small holes at the borders.

The cyborgification of reproductive processes became a feminist theme at the end of the twentieth century. Feminist anthropologists Lisa Mitchell and Eugenia Georges, in their coauthored essay "Cross-Cultural Cyborgs: Greek and Canadian Women's Discourses on Fetal Ultrasound," published in 1997, argue that the visualized fetus on the ultrasound screen is created through the merging of human and machine, what they call a "cyborg fetus." To support their argument, they draw on earlier work by Donna Haraway, who became well known in the 1980s for her celebration of the cyborg in her groundbreaking "A Manifesto for Cyborgs." However, Mitchell and Georges, in their 1997 essay, present a view of the cyborg that is different from Haraway's view. While Haraway's "Manifesto" embraces the cyborg's potential to help eliminate modern binaries between male and female, Mitchell and Georges argue instead that the ultrasound machine, when exerted on a fetus to assign it a sex, actually initiates processes of gendering even before birth.

After showing me her fetal scans, Louise asked if I could help her with something else at another time. I was curious to know what she had in mind but at first she wouldn't say. Then she told me, "You know I also work as a stage manager and soon I will decorate a film set with ultrasound machines. The actor plays the role of a pregnant woman." "Oh, how exciting," I answered and agreed to help her with the setting up of the ultrasound scene.

Before leaving the boutique, I took a photograph of Louise posing near the window display. "It's eye-catching," she said of the display. "Well, I hope it will bring in customers," I said and took another photograph of her. We said goodbye. I went outside and stood at the window looking in with Louise looking out at me. It was already dark outside, but I could see into her store window which was aglow with lights. But I was surprised when Louise suddenly lifted her shirt and showed me her bare pregnant belly, which I photographed through the glass. Then I took a lot of close-up pictures of her belly while playing around with the reflections and distortions created by the surface of the glass. On that same night I posted the photographs of Louise on the project website.

A few days later, Louise, who offered to give me all her fetal scans, told me she had enjoyed looking at the project website, especially at the photographs of her posing near the window display of her boutique. I didn't know it then, when I photographed her in that way, but I was partly following what Sandra Matthews and Laura Wexler (2000, 51) identify and describe as a "conventional middle-class motif." In their coauthored book *Pregnant Pictures* (2000), for which they collected and analyzed over 200 photographs of pregnancy taken in the United States from the late 1800s to the 1990s, Matthews and Wexler state that middle-class pregnant subjects have been depicted at a window more often than low-income pregnant subjects. The book examines photographs taken from obstetrical textbooks, childbirth manuals, advertisements for maternity clothes, public policy documents, fine art images, family snapshots, and media outlets. While examining this wide variety of photographs from diverse contexts, Matthews and Wexler (2000, 27) found that low-income pregnant subjects "are almost always pictured with other people in a social, often public, space, such as the street." By contrast, middle-class pregnant subjects are often photographed indoors, usually in a private and secure place, looking out a window.

One day I received a text message from Louise: "Could use your help again. Can you meet me tomorrow at the hospital where you placed your flyer?"

The next day I went to the hospital to meet Louise. I took the elevator to the second floor and found Louise in a room surrounded by ultrasound machines next to camera equipment. She was speaking to a film crew.

Louise, who also worked as a stage manager, was currently staging an ultrasound scene for a television movie. She rented ultrasound equipment for this scene but the shooting was already over now. "Sorry you missed it," she said. Looking around the room I was curious to know what had happened. She explained, "In this scene, where the actor plays a pregnant woman undergoing a prenatal exam, the ultrasound probe was placed on my belly. I myself didn't appear in the ultrasound scene but my fetus did. My fetus was in the camera frame on the ultrasound screen and it is now in this movie which will be shown on TV." Then Louise pointed to the ultrasound machines and asked me, "Could you roll them to the elevator and bring them downstairs for me?" Nodding my head, I started to move the machines. I thought, not only has she many fetal scans, she has also staged an ultrasound scene for a commercial film.

After the ultrasound machines were packed in the rental car, Louise said to me, "It's too bad you didn't get to see how we filmed today. But you could watch the movie when it appears on TV." I said okay and waved goodbye to Louise as she drove away with her ultrasound machines.

UNBORN SUBMARINES AND SUNKEN WINDOWS

In 1958, over sixty years ago, the first ultrasound images of a living fetus were published by the *Lancet*, one of the oldest and most renowned medical journals in the world. Appearing in the now classic article titled "Investigations of Abdominal Masses by Pulsed Ultrasound," these historical images were made in Glasgow under the supervision of the obstetrician Ian Donald, the leading figure in the development of prenatal technology. Donald (1969, 618) is famously quoted for having said, "There is not so much difference after all between a fetus in utero and a submarine at sea." With this statement Donald was referring to how ultrasound technology was initially used in naval warfare during the Second World War for underwater navigation. While the analogy between fetuses and submarines no longer exists today, it was once a theme in mainstream media. For example, in a feature story of *Life* magazine, published in 1965 under the title "A Sonar 'Look' at an Unborn Baby," the author writes: "The astonishing medical machine resting on this pregnant woman's abdomen in a Philadelphia hospital is 'looking' at her unborn child in precisely the same way a Navy surface ship homes in on enemy submarines [. . .] bombarding her with a beam of ultra-high-frequency sound waves" (Steinmann 1965, 45). The "enemy submarines" of which the author speaks were the German U-boats.

In the late 1970s, Germany was the first country in the world to make a fetal scan mandatory for all pregnancies without clinical indication (Erikson 2007, 188). As prenatal ultrasound became routine, it was no longer referred to in the media as a military defense weapon used to surveil submarines. "Ultrasound," as one medical text puts it, "provides a window of unsurpassed clarity into the gravid uterus" (Pretorius and Mahony 1990, 1, quoted in Mitchell 2001, 4). The word "window" conveys the idea of objectivity and is associated with glass, screen, perspective, display, frame, eye, light, photograph, canvas, and mirror (Friedberg 2006; Patterson 2011). Feminist scholars critique the frequent use of the word "window" in medical descriptions of fetal ultrasound images because it is a word that suggests a transparent and authentic view of the pregnant body, thereby obscuring the production of the image (Mitchell 2001; Boucher 2004; Roberts 2012). Also in anti-abortion propaganda, the word "window" is found for example in their oft-used slogan: "Fewer women would have abortions if wombs had windows" (see Ginsburg 1989, 104). Following the poststructuralist position of language as constructing rather than simply describing reality, in being called a window, the fetal ultrasound image is made into a window. Perceiving fetal scans as though they were windows to the fetus within the pregnant body is indeed a common cross-cultural experience in technologized societies (Mitchell 2001;

Boucher 2004; Roberts 2012). Some people not only look at the visualized fetus on the ultrasound screen; they also claim that the fetus smiles back at them (Roberts 2012, 67). For instance, British obstetrician Stuart Campbell (2006), who is a leading figure in the development of 3D and 4D ultrasound scanning techniques, has publicly stated that fetuses smile back at him when he performs ultrasound exams on his pregnant patients.

The medical metaphor of ultrasound as a transparent window providing objective evidence of fetal personhood can be contrasted with the window in contemporary artistic representations of pregnancy. Matthews and Wexler, in their book *Pregnant Pictures* (2000), discuss how the visual element of the window in the work of female photographers has been used to evoke the doubling of the pregnant body rather than the singularity of the fetus. As an example, Matthews and Wexler (2000, 51) analyze several pregnant self-portraits including Joan Harrison's "Ambivalence, July 2, 1997," in which the pregnant artist is shown "gazing out a window into the great unknown." As Matthews and Wexler point out, the artist's pregnant body blurs the boundaries between self and other, and between inside and outside, and in this sense, possesses the qualities of the window. Here, the window seems to encapsulate the blurring of body boundaries during pregnancy, possibly prompting viewers to reflect on the ambiguous nature of the pregnant body. This, I suggest, contrasts with the "window" of ultrasound, which visually isolates the fetus from the pregnant body and produces the fetus as an independent individual.

There are indeed different types of windows, each with their own literal and metaphoric meaning (Friedberg 2006). For example, the windows of a hospital serve to let in light and fresh air, which are the essential elements for life and good health. In a metaphorical sense, the large windows and glass facades of modern hospitals also symbolize class privilege in Western societies where "the more windows, the wealthier the owner" (Hauge 2015, 25). In the maternity wards of modern hospitals, nursery viewing windows offer a public view of newborns. The nursery viewing window, which is more of a glass wall along the hospital corridor near the delivery room, emerged in the early part of the twentieth century when the birthplace moved from homes to hospitals (Fagen 2017). At that time, the hospital standard was to separate an infant from its parent directly after the birth. The parent was supposed to recover in the delivery room while the infant was cared for by nurses in another room with a show window. The thick glass of the nursery viewing window was meant to function as a barrier to keep infections outside while also allowing parents to look at their newborns and to wave at them through sealed glass.

A HOME AND A FAMILY ALBUM

Maggie eventually got what she wanted: she gave birth in a good hospital with large glass windows. She was given a sanitized quiet room where she could rest the days before and after giving birth. One day after the birth, while Maggie was recovering, I went alone to the nursery viewing window. For a while I stood there, observing how the nurses took care of all the babies. The babies were wrapped tightly in soft blankets, arranged in rows of plastic bassinets. A few days later, Maggie left the hospital with her baby to go home to their new apartment. I felt happy for them.

Before the birth the apartment was still empty. On the day of the signing of the apartment lease, Maggie thanked me for finding the apartment, but she did not give me the fetal scan. Instead, she said, "We now need a bed to sleep on and a table to eat on." I could not say no even though I thought my job was done. So together we made a list of the things they needed to turn the apartment into a home. It wasn't just the big things; it was also the little things.

Even earlier, and before the birth, when I was helping her to set everything up for her new home, Maggie asked me, "Do you want to see the fetal scan?" I answered, "Of course, yes, please." She took out her wallet and there in her wallet was the fetal scan. I could see it half exposed in her wallet but not entirely and this bothered me. So, I asked Maggie when I could expect to get the fetal scan, how it was agreed upon, now that she got her apartment. She told me she would give me the fetal scan after the birth, which made me think she was more superstitious than she said she was.

The project became more complicated when Maggie said she didn't like how she appeared in certain photographs I had taken of her and posted on the project website. "I look sweaty and exhausted in them," she said. So, I reminded her that she had agreed to let herself be photographed and depicted on the project website.

The photographs that Maggie did not want to be shown were the ones that are typically omitted from the traditional family album. Maggie wanted to show only the photographs in which she was properly posing. Those were the ones in which she said she looked "normal." I answered, "It's not a question of people liking these photographs as with your Instagram posts. It's not about liking or not liking. That is not what matters in art. Art is supposed to pose questions and to be provocative."

To me the photographs in which Maggie looked stressed were the least staged and I felt it was important to show them because they captured the urgency of her unstable living situation. I was not convinced that the photographs she didn't "like" were not worth showing others. But after several discussions with Maggie, I had my doubts and removed some of the photographs from the project website. A few days later I looked at the altered version of the website and I saw that it had lost a certain quality. But I tried to accept this reworked version and subsequently sent a text message to Maggie asking for her opinion. After days of not hearing from her, Maggie called to say she was happy to see some photographs had been deleted from the website, but she wanted me to remove a few more.

Then there came the day Maggie gave me her fetal scan. I was curious to know if it was still in her wallet and it was. She opened her wallet as if to pay me and gave me her fetal scan as though it were money. I was a bit shocked to see her handle it like a payment, but all along that was what I had wanted to achieve, to receive a wage for my housework. It was a low-quality, blurry scan with lots of gray patches, taken with a standard 2D scanner. I put it in my wallet and thought, I have it now. Then I asked Maggie again what she thought of the project website, and she said she was still not pleased with it. So, I removed some more photographs and sent a text message to Maggie. After much texting back and forth, the content of the website was even more reduced.

It was now far from my original idea of creating an alternative website that challenged the enforced sacredness of the fetal scan by displacing it from the traditional family album. My intention behind the website was not only to defy the social convention of keeping the fetal scan as a keepsake, but also to interrogate the visual norm of smiling and posing in family photographs in general. But I could not communicate that to Maggie.

For the next few weeks, it gave me pleasure to keep the fetal scan in my wallet and to walk around with it. Sometimes I took it out and looked at it. I couldn't see a fetus or something like it, which was something I liked about it.

At a certain point during the days when I was walking around with the fetal scan in my wallet, I made the decision to deactivate the project website until the issue with the photographs was resolved. "I'll make it invisible, and it's only temporary," I wrote in an email to the project participants. The website remained hidden for months and I moved on to other projects. It was a gradual process but eventually I deleted the entire website, and the artistic fetal scan project was never again shown to a broader public. I abandoned the project altogether without knowing I would pick it up years later as part of my PhD thesis, titled "In a Quick Sketch of a Fetus." To write this autoethnographic essay—here, I have drawn from and build upon existing research undertaken for "In a Quick Sketch of a Fetus," where the artistic fetal scan project was analyzed among other projects (see Gonzalez Suero 2022b).

As I've reflected in this autoethnography on the artistic fetal scan project, I've become more aware of how I thought it was up to me—the artist—to decide what the project should look like. I can see in retrospect that there was a lack of clarity between me and Maggie, for whom the kind of socially engaged art practice that she agreed to take part in was unfamiliar. But with the pressure of having to find the apartment before the birth, there was no time for us to discuss the photographs I was taking. I also realize that Maggie as an African woman has probably had to work hard to be accepted as a "good mother" in the German context which can still be hostile toward people of color. I can therefore understand why Maggie wanted me to depict her in a "normal" way, in accordance with society's current image of a "good mother," which feminist scholarship shows is one of being in control (see, for example, Tyler 2011). It was our different views regarding the photographs of the project, not the hardships that we experienced during the project itself, that maybe steered the project toward its non-visual form.

NOTES

1. Names have been changed to protect identities.
2. The project website no longer exists for reasons discussed in this chapter.

REFERENCES

Beharry, Shruti, and Michael Heinrich. 2018. "Is the Hype around the Reproductive Health Claims of Maca (*Lepidium meyenii* Walp.) Justified?" *Journal of Ethnopharmacology* 211 (January): 126–170. http://dx.doi.org/10.1016/j.jep.2017.08.003.

Boucher, Joanne. 2004. "Ultrasound: A Window to the Womb?: Obstetric Ultrasound and the Abortion Rights Debate." *Journal of Medical Humanities* 25, no. 1 (Spring): 7–19.

Bridges, Khiara M. 2011. *Reproducing Race: An Ethnography of Pregnancy as a Site of Racialization*. Berkeley, CA: University of California Press.

Campbell, Stuart. 2006. "Don't Tear a Smiling Foetus From the Womb." *The Telegraph*, October 4, 2006. http://www.telegraph.co.uk/comment/personal-view/3632855/Dont-tear-a-smiling-foetus-from-the-womb.html.

Donald, Ian, John MacVicar, and Tom G. Brown. 1958. "Investigation of Abdominal Masses by Pulsed Ultrasound." *Lancet* 271, no. 7032 (June): 1188–1195. https://doi.org/10.1016/S0140-6736(58)91905-6.

Donald, Ian. 1969. "On Launching a New Diagnostic Science." *American Journal of Obstetrics and Gynecology* 103, no. 5 (March): 609–628.

Duden, Barbara. 1993. *Disembodying Women: Perspectives on Pregnancy and the Unborn*. Translated by Lee Hoinacki. Cambridge, MA: Harvard University Press.

Ellis, Carolyn. 1991. "Sociological Introspection and Emotional Experience." *Symbolic Interaction* 14, no. 1 (Spring): 23–50. https://doi.org/10.1525/si.1991.14.1.23.

Ellis, Carolyn. 2004. *The Ethnographic I: A Methodological Novel about Autoethnography.* New York: AltaMira Press.

Ellis, Carolyn. 2008. "Systematic Sociological Introspection." In *The Sage Encyclopedia of Qualitative Research Methods*, edited by Lisa M. Given, 853–854. Thousand Oaks, CA: Sage. https://doi.org/10.4135/9781412963909.n443.

Erikson, Susan L. 2001. "Maternity Care Policies and Maternity Care Practices: A Tale of Two Germanies." In *Birth by Design: Pregnancy, Maternity Care, and Midwifery in North America and Europe*, edited by Raymond De Vries, Cecilia Benoit, Edwin van Teijlingen, and Sirpa Wrede, 203–217. London and New York: Routledge.

Erikson, Susan L. 2007. "Fetal Views: Histories and Habits of Looking at the Fetus in Germany." *Journal of Medical Humanities* 28 (October): 187–212. https://doi.org/10.1007/s10912-007-9040-2.

Erikson, Susan L. 2015. "Interview with Prof. Dr. Susan Erikson (Senior Fellow)." Interview by Yanda Bango, Ratanak Khun, and Diana León-Espinoza. *Kate Hamburger Kolleg's Interns Project*, March 25, 2015. https://internsproject.wordpress.com/2015/03/25/interview-to-prof-dr-susan-erikson-senior-fellow-2/.

Fagen, Hannah. 2017. "Handmaids, Hospitals, and the Pageantry of the Newborn Nursery Window." *Nursing Clio*, July 20, 2017. https://nursingclio.org/2017/07/20/handmaids-hospitals-and-the-pageantry-of-the-newborn-nursery-window/.

Federici, Silvia. 1975. *Wages against Housework.* Bristol: Power of Women Collective and Falling Wall Press.

Federici, Silvia. 2008. "Witch-Hunting, Globalization, and Feminist Solidarity in Africa Today." *Journal of International Women's Studies* 10, no. 1 (October): 21–35.

Franklin, Sarah. 1997. *Embodied Progress: A Cultural Account of Assisted Conception.* London and New York: Routledge.

Friedberg, Anne. 2006. *The Virtual Window: From Alberti to Microsoft.* Cambridge, MA: The MIT Press.

Ginsburg, Faye D. 1989. *Contested Lives: The Abortion Debate in an American Community.* Berkeley, CA: University of California Press.

Gonzales, Gustavo F. 2012. "Ethnobiology and Ethnopharmacology of *Lepidium meyenii* (Maca), a Plant from the Peruvian Highlands." *Evidence-Based Complementary and Alternative Medicine* (October 2, 2011): 1–10. https://doi.org/10.1155/2012/193496.

Gonzalez Suero, Anna. 2022a. "The Foetus Phallus Studio." In *Performing the Penis: Phalluses in 21st Century Cultures*, edited by Meredith Jones and Evelyn Callahan, 26–47. London and New York: Routledge. https://doi: 10.4324/9781003108481-3.

Gonzalez Suero, Anna. 2022b. "In a Quick Sketch of a Fetus." PhD diss., Goldsmiths, University of London.

Hauge, Bettina. 2015. "Window Stories: The Significance of Windows to Germans—A Qualitative, Anthropological Investigation of Qualities of a Window." Kongens Lyngby, Denmark: DTU Management Engineering.

Kapsalis, Terri. 1997. *Public Privates: Performing Gynecology from Both Ends of the Speculum.* Durham and London: Duke University Press.

Knecht, Michi, Maren Klotz, and Stefan Beck, eds. 2012. *Reproductive Technologies as Global Form: Ethnographies of Knowledge, Practices, and Transnational Encounters*. Frankfurt and New York: Campus Verlag.

Leavitt, Judith W. 1986. *Brought to Bed: Childbearing in America, 1750–1950*. New York: Oxford University Press.

Matthews, Sandra, and Laura Wexler. 2000. *Pregnant Pictures*. New York and London: Routledge.

Mitchell, Lisa M. 2001. *Baby's First Picture: Ultrasound and the Politics of Fetal Subjects*. Toronto: University of Toronto Press. https://doi.org/10.3138/9781442671140.

Mitchell, Lisa M., and Eugenia Georges. 1997. "Cross-Cultural Cyborgs: Greek and Canadian Women's Discourses on Fetal Ultrasound." *Feminist Studies* 23, no. 2 (Summer), 373–401.

Patterson, Duncan. 2011. "'There's Glass Between Us': A Critical Examination of 'the Window' in Art and Architecture from Ancient Greece to the Present Day." *FORUM Ejournal* 10 (June): 1–21.

Petchesky, Rosalind P. 1987. "Fetal Images: The Power of Visual Culture in the Politics of Reproduction." *Feminist Studies* 13, no. 2 (Summer): 263–292. https://doi.org/10.2307/3177802.

Prescott, Heather Munro. 2003. "'Guides to Womanhood': Gynaecology and Adolescent Sexuality in the Post–Second World War Era." In *Women, Health, and Nation: Canada and the United States since 1945*, edited by Georgina Feldberg, Molly Ladd-Taylor, Alison Li, and Kathryn McPherson, 199–222. Montreal: McGill-Queen's University.

Pretorius, Jack D., and Barry S. Mahoney. 1990. "The Role of Obstetrical Ultrasound." In *Diagnostic Ultrasound of Fetal Anomalies: Text and Atlas*, edited by David A. Nyberg, Barry S. Mahony, and Jack D. Pretorius, 1–20. Chicago: Year Book Medical Publishers.

Roberts, Julie. 2012. *The Visualised Foetus: A Cultural and Political Analysis of Ultrasound Imagery.* Farnham: Ashgate.

Samerski, Silja. 2011. "Genetic Counseling and the Fiction of Choice: Taught Self-Determination as a New Technique of Social Engineering." In *Between Self-Determination and Social Technology: Medicine, Biopolitics and the New Techniques of Procedural Management*, edited by Katrin Braun, 95–125. Bielefeld: Transcript.

Samerski, Silja. 2015. *The Decision Trap: Genetic Education and Its Social Consequences*. Exeter, UK: Imprint Academic.

Sandelowski, Margarete. 2000. "This Most Dangerous Instrument: Property, Power, and the Vaginal Speculum." *Journal of Obstetric, Gynecologic and Neonatal Nursing* 29, no. 1 (January/February): 73–82. https://doi:10.1111/j.1552-6909.2000.tb02759.x.

Sänger, Eva. 2015. "Obstetrical Care as a Matter of Time: Ultrasound Screening, Temporality and Prevention." *History and Philosophy of the Life Sciences* 37, no. 1: 105–120. https://doi.org/10.1007/s40656-014-0056-4.

Sasson, Vanessa R., and Jane Marie Law, eds. 2009. *Imagining the Fetus: The Unborn in Myth, Religion, and Culture*. New York: Oxford University Press. https://doi:10.1093/acprof:oso/9780195380040.001.0001.

Steinmann, Marion. 1965. "A Sonar 'Look' at an Unborn Baby." *LIFE* 58, no. 2 (January 15, 1965): 45–46.

Tyler, Imogen. 2011. "Pregnant Beauty: Maternal Femininities under Neoliberalism." In *New Femininities: Postfeminism, Neoliberalism and Subjectivity*, edited by Rosalind Gill and Christina Scharff, 21–36. Basingstoke and New York: Palgrave Macmillan.

Weeks, Kathi. 2011. *The Problem With Work: Feminism, Marxism, Antiwork Politics, and Postwork Imaginaries*. Durham and London: Duke University Press.

Whiteley, Rebecca. 2023. *Birth Figures: Early Modern Prints and the Pregnant Body*. Chicago: University of Chicago Press.

Chapter 4

The Alterlife of Disabled Fetal Imaginaries

Understanding Irradiation and Disability after New Reproductive Technologies

Misria Shaik Ali

MC Palle and Kottala are villages located atop the uranium ore belt in the Indian State of Andhra Pradesh. As someone who has borne witness to the slow processes of the residents of MC Palle and Kottala becoming irradiated, Shiva [name changed] was advised by M. Srinath Reddy, former local government authority and leader of the Uranium Workers Union to accompany my visits to contaminated farms. Stuck between an ethnographer who cannot speak Telugu and an irradiated village that he cares for, Shiva uses sticky words, in the limited English he knows, to explain involuntary childlessness as a condition of becoming irradiated in the age of New Reproductive Technologies (NRT). He said,

> *Diseases—one by one starting*, madam . . . Now we have a few diseases—body pain, cancer, body itching, stomach pains, pimples on cow . . . also, abortion, we can't say how many more *diseases* are to come! We need to think about what the *future problems* would be. In a [Telugu actor] Rajasekhar *movie*, they show that in *uranium places*, there are *handicapped children* around—they are *visible*! Presently, in *MC Palle village*, there are no *handicapped children*. Reason being, many *face abortions* within *three months* of conception. Plus, *legs* are showing *no growth* and *hands* are showing *no growth*, so they are being medically advised to undergo abortion. So, *handicap-ers* are just not made visible. Today we have a lot of *technologies*, they do *scanning* in *three months* and

> say there is *no leg growth, or another body part* has not grown, *so abortion. Ten years back*, there was no such *technologies*. In *uranium affected places* like *Jadugoda and Jharkhand*, there are many *handicapped children* because there was *no technology* and they are also poor people, they have no amount for expensive technology. [I have emphasized the English words spoken in the interview; Ramanjaneyulu and Shiva, *Interview,* October 22, 2021]

Shiva simultaneously constructs "disability" as a sign of "radioactive contamination" and "environmental damage" reinforcing the double bind of disability: "the disabled body is necessary to give risk . . . any meaning, and yet [such constructions demand that] the disabled body must remain invisible" (Ray 2017; Mannur 2017). During the initial days of my research in MC Palle and Kottala, villages in YSR District, Andhra Pradesh, India, as a theorist, I had a lot of questions running through my mind: "Why do my ethnographic subjects lack an eco-crip perspective?" With a fear of a complex situation at Tummalapalle I asked myself, "Why is disability undesirable for them?" "Can the subaltern speak?" "Can I intervene as an ethnographer to build such a consciousness or simply document the irony of the subaltern?" My inner voice said, "Enlighten them!"

Shiva spoke to me about the relations between NRT, medically induced abortions, and the visibility of radioactive exposure that compose involuntary childlessness at MC Palle and Kottala when Shiva and I were at Ramanjaneyulu's farm to learn about his experiments with radioporosity (Shaik Ali 2023). The soil at Ramanjaneyulu's farm has been soaking in the irradiated water with a concentration of 690 uranium particles per billion (ppb) at least since 2016 when farmers first noticed water contamination on their lands. With the curiosity to understand how irradiated water interacts with soil, crops, and wind, he has developed techniques on "radioporosity" to live, grow, and do the barely sustainable agriculture on his irradiated land (Shaik Ali 2023). After several interviews with farmers and families of involuntary childlessness and disabled children, I observed that for people enduring environmental injustice, disability justice is a matter of everyday practice and not begging of a theoretical intervention by an outsider ethnographer like myself—their lives are "already-altered" by their chemical relations (Murphy 2017). As "alter-collectivities" that painfully embody death and destruction as outcomes of "environmental violence," they engender the "capacity to become otherwise" (Murphy 2017). Their altered practices and demands recognize that "colonial and environmental violence have already happened"[1] and have entered through the porous spaces between their lives and the nuclear-industrial complex, even as science and social science research merely presses on how to contain radiation within the complex.

Scholarship that analyzes the difficulty in attributing genetic effects (Hayakeyama 2022), reproductive health issues (Folkers 2022), kidney issues, cancer, and lungs to low- level exposure (Creager 2015), radium (Clark 2000), depleted and natural uranium (Abraham 2012), and radon (Rennie 2005) unravels the historical, social, cultural, and transnational politics of nuclear safety standards setting. Such incisive works highlight that the history of standard-setting and experimentation in radiation protection are as complex as the scientific attribution of the cause of health effects to ongoing (nuclear) industrial contamination (Hecht 2012; Boudia et al. 2018; Creager 2018; Mitchell 2022). Their conclusions directly or indirectly problematize industries employing contested scientific standards and highlight how their employability dilutes accountability to further industrial agenda. However, as an STS ethnographer, when I saw people *becoming irradiated* at MC Palle and Kottala, the scientific (also, social scientific) interest in studying siloed health effects (like genetic effects, cancer, or dermatitis) of the siloed radioactive exposures seemed futile. The focus on "becoming irradiated" shifts the ontological focus from bodies caught at the interstices of safety standards and categories of nuclear regulation that aim to control and contain irradiation. Becoming irradiated as a ruination science (Ureta 2020) alters the ontological focus on the nuclear containment, treating radiation as that which has never been successfully controlled "enough" (Wellock 2021). It remedies the increasing trend in social scientific studies to employ categories like "nuclear safety" and "safety standards" as objects of study as they are paradoxically determined by matters of concern to nuclear science. It is committed to complex and compounded health and environmental realities and futures of irradiated places, refusing to hold at the center of the analysis "nuclear safety"—"a very much simpler" means to "radiation protection" (IAEA 2007).

As radiation leaves the nuclear containment (as it does always and everywhere) even as they are instrumented with control systems of nuclear safety, it forges chemical relations with bodies and with other chemicals that complexifies contamination and disease causation (Burch 2019). As causational claims are muffled by official statements like "may be due to [this reason or that]," irradiation reproduces new governance modalities of attribution that stop at "maybe" diverging from industrial accountability for the harm caused. This paper delivers nuanced relational engagements between nuclear-environmental and health regulatory authorities and industries around TUMM in an effort to critically position the contaminated environment in debates around social impacts of medical technologies bringing together disability, women's reproductive and environmental justice.

In the first section of the chapter, I demonstrate the emergence of new governance techniques that diffuses the responsibility for protection of health and environment from irradiation through divisible governance (Howey and Naele 2022) and what I call "layered" risk governance at MC Palle and Kottala. In these irradiated spaces, radioactive contamination is multiple ["may be due to" multiple causes] but never unclear for those enduring radiation violence even as they remain invisible on official registers. As people become irradiated and their bodies come to bear radiation's effects, I analyze how the new nuclear and environmental governance model weakens decentralized health governance in the area while strengthening private healthcare. This chapter talks about the emergence of the nuclear-medical-industrial complex at TUMM that through new nuclear, environmental, and health governance diffuses accountability and creates parasitical relationships among the actors involved. Through an analysis of employee monitoring, reproductive masculinity (Daniels 2006), female reproductive health, and the use of disabled fetal imagery (Rapp 2000), I show how nuclear and medical experts shape the production of normate bodies (Garland-Thomson 1996) and compulsory able-bodiedness (McRuer 2017) leading to involuntary childlessness in contaminated places watched over by NRT. Against this, through the relational model of disability (Kafer 2013), I expound the alterlife positionality of the families of involuntary childlessness and the villagers that critiques both compulsory able-bodiedness and uncritical mutant optimism that unintentionally capitalizes the pain of disability (Masco 2004; Kriskey 2020, 21).

This chapter is developed from my sensory and multispecies ethnographic fieldwork at MC Palle and Kottala in September and October 2021 with the aid of Dr. K. Babu Rao, a retired scientist with Human Rights Forum, M. Srinath Reddy, a local Tamil-speaking translator, a local Hindi-speaking translator, and a friend who volunteers to translate and accompany my visit. I interviewed farmers, villagers, and women in groups, namely *Racchabanda*,[2] and conducted one-on-one interviews with consent. I also conducted two focus group interviews with women facing menstrual and reproductive health issues for 3 hours each. In these interviews, I specifically attended to how people came to know radioactive contamination in their villages through sensing effects on human and more-than-human bodies including water and air.

MAY BE TUMM'S ENVIRONMENT AND NUCLEAR GOVERNANCE, OR MAY NOT *BE*!

At Tummalapalle Uranium Mine and Mill (TUMM), over 2,350 tonnes of uranium ore are mined, crushed, and processed through an alkali leaching process to procure 1,350 grams of uranium. The residual waste of 73,000 tonnes as irradiated sludge consisting of over 19 chemicals is deposited through a system of five pipes every month in a 956-hectare pond-like structure called the tailing pond (about 3 miles from the mine). The tailing pond is an impoundment technology of uranium milling and mining processes. It is lined with materials stipulated by regulatory authorities to ensure that the chemical slurry, or "tailings" do not seep into the underground aquifers. The lining should be designed in a way to ensure effective containment of tailings within the pond so that residents of the MC Palle and Kottala village hamlets and the agricultural farms around the tailing pond are protected from the radioactive harms of UCIL's operations.[3] Some of the farms in the area are as old as 200 years. Eight years ago, farming and agriculture made the villagers, some of whom also happen to be relatives of the state's Chief Minister Jagan Mohan Reddy, richer than many urban upper-middle-class families in India.[4] But now, the farm income is dwindling against increased medical expenditure. The villagers' attribute their livelihood struggles to the inadequate lining of the mine's tailing pond. Due to inadequate (yet, "safe") lining, the radioactive tailing materials have been leaking into the underground aquifers plausibly since 2012 when TUMM began its operations in the region.

In 2016, some agricultural landowners observed that the water in their land had turned white and that it tasted salty. After a few others faced losses of about USD 25,000,[5] the farmers sent water samples from their agricultural borewells to a centrally recognized laboratory with the help of ex–panchayat leader and the region's Uranium Workers Union (UWU) leader, M. Srinath Reddy. The result showed uranium concentrations in water samples ranging from 40.35 to 405.32 particles per billion (ppb) and the farmers enrolled the district magistrate, state agricultural department, and the Andhra Pradesh Pollution Control Board (APPCB) to evaluate the situation.[6] The three regulatory organizations that were involved are jurisdictionally distinct[7]—district magistrate-cum-district collector as an appointed civil servant is responsible for the district's law and order and revenue administration respectively; the APPCB is a state-level pollution control authority that falls under the Ministry of Environmental, Forest and Climate Change that is headed by an elected representative; the state agriculture department cooperates with the Ministry of Agriculture and Farmers Welfare, also headed by an elected representative. Furthermore, these departments are distinct from and operate outside of the Department of Atomic Energy (DAE) and India's Atomic Energy Regulatory Board (AERB), both of which are under the Atomic Energy Commission of India (AECI). Uranium Corporation of India Limited (UCIL) is a public sector undertaking under the DAE and its operations at uranium industries like TUMM are regulated by AERB, which recommends and monitors nuclear safety standards. The contamination brought these jurisdictionally district organizations into relations and M. Srinath Reddy, a democratically upheld extra-governmental village authority, frequently communicated with these authorities about the contamination.

The APPCB and agricultural department, after multiple tests and field visits where they spoke to villagers, came to a conclusion that the agricultural lands are affected by radioactive contamination.[8] The APPCB issued a notice to UCIL asking it to show the cause of "690 to 4000" uranium ppb in agricultural borewells as "against the permissible limit of 60 ppb" (APPCB 2007). It alleged that UCIL did not line the tailing pond with a polyethylene sheet as stipulated by APPCB when it issued its consent for UCIL to establish the mine. UCIL simply said that the lining it had provided with clay met the "AERB [safety] guidelines" for [im]permeability and so UCIL "felt" that the polyethylene layer [as recommended by APPCB] was not "necessary" as "an extra precautionary measure" (APPCB 2019). While the AERB stipulations address nuclear safety or the safeness of nuclear operations and technologies, those recommended by APPCB concern control of pollution. Layering the tailing pond's ground surface was then an act of "layered governance"[9] where pollution and nuclear safety stipulations provided by distinct governmental bodies, APPCB and AERB respectively, are layered on top of each other to conform with the distinct regulatory jurisdictions of these bodies. However, UCIL simply overlooked pollution control stipulations, namely polyethylene lining, by stating that it had followed nuclear safety guidelines, namely clay, to attain the desired impermeability.[10] Impressed by the need to align its practices with the rhetoric of "nuclear energy is safe" (as in, safely designed), UCIL practiced divisible governance, justified the safeness of the lining through AERB safety guidelines, and thereby was solely driven only by nuclear safety concerns.

The wider concern here is how governance techniques like nuclear safety shape the phenomenon of radiation (contamination) being invisible.[11] Simply put, nuclear safety, more than a "scientific" technique that makes nuclear energy actually safe, is primarily a governance technique that is used to render radioactive contamination visible or invisible. When APPCB questioned UCIL about inadequate lining and the consequent permeability, UCIL substantiated its claim about the lining's impermeability as it aligns with the "AERB [safety] guidelines." UCIL also further substantiated impermeability by pointing to their radiation monitoring techniques in the area to check possible contamination like the borewells that are dug by UCIL deep into the ground to collect water samples. In its show-cause response, UCIL added that the sample collected from such monitoring borewells did not show any abnormal levels of uranium concentration confirming "no migration of pollutants . . . to surrounding aquifers" (APPCB 2019). When APPCB stated that the monitoring borewells are in an uncontaminated region (north of the tailing pond) and inquired as to who decided their location, UCIL stated that the location was decided "as per AERB [safety] guidelines" (Pranesh 2018). After dislodging its responsibility by pointing to safety guidelines, UCIL stated that the uranium contamination in agricultural borewells found in APPCB's test *may be* due to the "varied concentration of in-situ uranium content in rock" or simply put, contamination is due to naturally occurring radiation and "not anthropogenic" (Government of India & Department of Atomic Energy PSU section, 2022).[12] Whereas APPCB pointed to baseline values of radiation before the establishment of the mine and said that "the reasons for increase of concentrations of Uranium to manifold *may be* due to the following reasons: the lining of TP is not proper; the locations of monitoring borewells are not correct and hence they are not representing the true nature of groundwater . . . " (APPCB 2018).

Both APPCB and UCIL resorted to arriving at the cause of irradiation through probability—"maybe" due to inadequate lining and monitoring (in APPCB's response) versus "maybe" due to in-situ uranium content in rock (in UCIL's response). APPCB demanded UCIL to reply with "documentary evidence" and "scientific evidence" that the contamination is not due to its operations and is, only, radiation pollution (APPCB 2018). As for scientific evidence, UCIL pointed out that it has followed safe design and monitoring and dislocated its accountability without further scientific studies and documentary evidence like newer underground hydrogeological mapping. While irradiation itself was made visible, the accountability for it was contested as UCIL had followed the nuclear safety guidelines and through the scientism of what I call the nuclear safety episteme. UCIL's responses gain its legitimacy from the "nuclear safety episteme"—when nuclear technologies are designed, operated, and maintained safely, it will result in radiation protection, or the protection of health and the environment from irradiation. However, nuclear safety does not always lead to radiation protection and the scientism encasing the nuclear safety episteme helps in diffusing the nuclear industry's accountability. It divides the accountability for radiation risks between the APPCB and AERB jurisdictions that ensure pollution control and nuclear regulation.

By dividing risks among varied governance authorities, the cause of irradiation in the area was up in the air and radiation in the environment seeped into human bodies through porous boundaries; human and non-human in MC Palle and Kottala came to bear the effects of radiation exposure on the body. In places where the source of radioactive contamination is acknowledged like Chernobyl, "the pain and suffering [of radiation victims] are rationalized" into authentic "social instruments" to measure the scale of industrial harm and negotiate policy practices and compensation producing biological citizenship (Petryna 2013, 14–15). Whereas in places like the Androy region in Madagascar, where women were employed in sorting uranium ore and the exposures were the norm, the absence of bodily effects does not automatically translate to absence of "danger" (Hecht 2012). Nuclear scholar Gabrielle Hecht asks, "If women remained fertile [that is, without bodily effects], perhaps there was no danger after all?" (225). However, in places like MC Palle and Kottala, there is no regulatory monitoring and messaging of radiation doses absorbed by bodies as the harms are supposedly contained through safety measures like tailing pond lining, and the source of harms that are borne by bodies are diffused by a politics of "maybe" affecting demands for state and polluter's compensation. So, here, radiation exposure is known through bodily effects only and not through usual nuclear scientific units like the roentgen (unit for radiation traveling through air), rad (unit for the amount of radiation deposited in materials as they pass), or msv (dose equivalent that is the amount of radiation absorbed combined with the medical effects of that type of radiation). Without any measure or message, in the biosocial registers of becoming irradiated (where there is no recognition of contamination or accountability for it), bodily effects are people's own version of dose equivalent. As Srinath Reddy explains,

> The main problem is, they [the villagers] cannot directly know radiation. They cannot see radiation. That's why they complain about what they see. Water, that's something they can see. If he takes a bath, he has a reaction. Immediately he can observe and say that water is different. They cannot say anything about radiation. The effect and impact are cancer. (*Racchabanda, Interview,* September 24, 2021)

Bodies bearing such effects without recognition of the cause of harm meant that these bodies could not rigidify their illness-based identities as victims of uranium mining and mill and so they were constrained to collectivize against UCIL as "biological citizens" (Petryna 2013). They were left with convoluted responses embedded in neoliberal and new governance techniques of addressing radioactive harms that decitizenizes and dehumanizes their radioactive subjectivities. While denying its role in irradiation of bodies, UCIL, as a matter of its good intentions to demonstrate "its care for environment and social issues," set up RO water plants for "providing safe drinking water in surrounding villages" under its Corporate Social Responsibility (CSR) project (UCIL and Mecon Ltd. 2020). Ultimately, as the enactment of layered and divisible risk governance operationalizes new governance models the locus of regulatory authority remains diffused "among governmental agencies, private actors such as NGOs, and regulated companies themselves," complicating industrial accountability for environmental harms (Conley and Williams 2005). Conley and Williams state that the problem of representation and accountability in new governance models is also abundant in the CSR movement, making CSR an "exercise" of "the new governance" model (Conley and Williams 2005). The new governance model concretized through layered and divisible governance techniques shaped how the public and private health authorities recorded and responded to radiation's effects on women's reproductive health (explored in the next section). As health governance deferred its own accountability for public health monitoring and redressal, in the next section, I analyze how MC Palle and Kottala villagers are forced into parasitical relationship with TUMM to respond to their burgeoning medical expenditure, making TUMM a nuclear-medical-industrial complex. Even as (the cause of) contamination *may be* multiple, never unclear, I observed that the reproductive capacities are activated to align with a nationalist imaginary of healthy and productive citizens under the duress of nuclear and NRT engendering biopolitics without biological citizenship (Rapp 2000).

TUMM'S NUCLEAR-MEDICAL-INDUSTRIAL COMPLEX

The agitation at MC Palle and Kottala villages against TUMM began in the 1990s when UCIL started to acquire agricultural lands for setting up TUMM. The villagers agreed to give consent for the project after the former prime minister Y. S. Rajashekhara Reddy assured that every family would receive employment and monetary compensation (Interview with Srinath Reddy, September 23, 2021). However, UCIL has, arguably, only provided compensation to those agricultural landowners whose lands have been acquired for the construction of TUMM's facilities and they are colloquially referred to as "land-losers." Since the 2018 contamination, farmers and village residents say that "although we did not lose land to UCIL's construction, we have lost our lands to [TUMM's contaminating] operations. So, we want UCIL to see us as land-losers, take our [residential and agricultural] land and give us money and employment. We will leave the village." UCIL's permanent employees are covered under corporate medical insurance which is not available to other villagers who are facing similar health issues. To understand their sense of belonging, I asked, "But these farms are inherited from your grandfathers. Are you connected to your village or land?" They immediately stopped me, "We will die ma'am! We will die drinking this water. . . . At least we need to *protect* our kids and future generations and need medical insurance" (*Racchabanda,* September 24, 2021).

Villagers widely assume that the only way to treat the health ailments is through the medical insurance that employment at UCIL assures, creating a situation of parasitical codependency salient to mining communities (Sikina 2022). Triggered by the trauma of my own codependent relations, I told many villagers, "But as citizens, you are entitled to clean air and water." Many villagers laughed, a few sighed, and others simply rolled their eyes at my naivete. A farming couple who, having faced three back-to-back spontaneous abortions, angrily said, "We want UCIL to leave" (*Interview,* October 18, 2021). I asked, "But people in your village want UCIL to stay to get employment and insurance. Shouldn't it be the government that remediates your soil and addresses your health effects?" The husband replied, "They [government] have not even kept their promises [of compensation and employment]. How are we to believe they will remediate our soil or take care of us?" (*Interview,* October 18, 2021). His emotions placed "the imperiled body" and the land at "the center of [his] eroding trust" in the state that has wounded his belongingness to the state (Zaretsky 2018, 12). Nuclear scholar Natasha Zaretsky analyzes how the Three Mile Island (TMI) conservative response to ecological disaster led to a "patriotic body politics" where the imperiled irradiated body and fetus were used to further distrust in the "government as it had turned against those who had been most loyal to it." This wounded belongingness would return as a belief in the nuclear safety episteme when I discuss about medically insured UCIL employees at the end of this section. As my interlocuter interrupted and said, "In the current situation, it's best if they stay so they can get medical insurance." The lack of governmental attention and care to public health has conditioned the villagers to accept forced displacement and the regulated industry's corporate medical insurance as measures to mitigate the consequences of radiation exposure on health. Thereby, the mitigation of radioactive exposures are not operationalized through instruments of nuclear safety but through the new environmental-health governance model of TUMM's nuclear-medico-industrial complex. The villagers turn to M. Srinath Reddy for making their suffering heard.[13]

Alter-ing TUMM's Social Movement

On the first day of my preliminary interview, September 24, 2021, I spoke to some farmers in the area to understand how they sensed and understood radiation and contamination and Srinath Reddy was translating the farmers' words. Shortly after, Srinath Reddy went over to speak with women villagers while I continued to talk to the male farmers with my translator. On the way back to Srinath Reddy's house on the barely lit UCIL mine roads, he told me:

> Until now, I targeted only those farmers who lost land to UCIL. Those who were not getting jobs [or money to compensate for their lost land as promised by authorities], I concentrated on that. [Further,] on cultivable lands where borewells [were] contaminated by UCIL, I gave importance to which farmer and agricultural lands where the contaminated borewells are. I never thought about women in the village . . . [abortion] their problems. We had cancer cases but [I] estimated only employees' families were affected [by diseases] initially. Now a

lot of people inside the village who are not employees are also affected. (Srinath Reddy, *interview,* October 16, 2021)

In the front yard of the agitation against contamination at MC Palle and Kottala, the primary concerns were the lining of the tailing pond and monetary or job compensation for lands acquired by UCIL. At this moment, the words from my dissertation literature review, written pre-COVID in March 2020, flashed: while India's nuclear scholarship extensively analyzes concerns of dissent, citizenship (health and environmental impacts), labor and land relations in nuclear development, mirroring concerns of old left, the biomedical construction of radiation at the intersection of gender, caste, religion, human/nonhuman divide, race, etc.[14] are yet to receive sufficient attention in nuclear scholarship in/of India. As Srinath Reddy expressed that his care had expanded, the dark UCIL mine roads merged with the Kadapa-Pulivendula Road where the CM Jagan Mohan Reddy's residence is located. The CM visits his residence once a year, and within 10 minutes, we reached Srinath's house from the CM's ancestral home. During dinner, he said in a disturbed voice, "Misria, you need to conduct a focus group for women of the village to understand all the women issues [like abortion, menstrual cycles, etc]." In Srinath Reddy's words, I sensed a shift to go beyond labor and land politics of nuclear development to include the gendered effects of irradiation into the struggle, that is, a movement from old left to new left in TUMM's irradiation movement.

"Women issues" have, however, never left the backyard of their contaminated houses, where "women, because they do a lot of household work. do dishes, cook and wash clothes, use more of the contaminated water," exposing them to radiation differentially (Anjali, *Interview*, October 17, 2021).[15] The water that MC Palle women use is from the municipal borewell that was found to contain 265.12 uranium ppb in March 2018. Anjali says that the reason why women face the effects of radiation more is due to the gendered household roles at MC Palle village, and points to the biosocial life of radioactive contamination in MC Palle. As the productive source of male bodies of 18–35 years mobilized towards indigenous nuclear energy production[16] at TUMM, only their bodies are monitored for dose equivalent. It ensures the health of those bodies that are used to further the nation's nuclear productivity, development, and aspiration. As the health governance in the region is carried out through occupational safety regulation and corporate employment benefits, women's bodies that are often exposed to contaminated water are overlooked in radiation monitoring. Such a regulatory oversight delineates bodies "unproductive" for the atomic state as unworthy of radiation monitoring and marks "women" who "satisfy the water needs of their families and society" outside of "productive labour," leading to nuclear "maldevelopment"

(Shiva 1988). Ecofeminist Vandana Shiva marks development that is "bereft of the feminine" production (in households) in the nation's productive capacity as maldevelopment (4). Such gendered social relations define and shape knowledge made about radiation contamination. When women are involved in the process of making knowledge production about radiation and its effect, they fight the invisibility of radiation and their own invisibility as knowledge producers in the society, as in the case of Fukushima (Kimura 2016; Sklyar 2019) and in TMI (Zaretsky 2018).

New Health Governance

Women in MC Palle and Kottala, as I demonstrate below, are rendered vulnerable by the (orchestrated) invisibility of radiation compounded by socio-technical vulnerabilities—firstly, the nuclear safety episteme[17] binds women to understand radiation's visibility through bodily effects like menstrual issues, spontaneous abortion, and fetal growth; secondly, gendered understandings of reproductive health issues as "women issues" and the reproductive masculinity; thirdly, their social position to make knowledge as women that is, fourthly, compounded by the construction of villagers as lay, and nuclear and medical authorities as experts.[18] A woman who faced spontaneous abortion said,

> When I faced spontaneous abortion, I was 6 weeks into my pregnancy. But my spontaneous abortion was not counted. My sense is that local health workers are instructed to only count women who face spontaneous abortions after 90 days of pregnancy. The health department skews the record through such instructions. Most people face abortion within 30–60 days.

To facilitate India's local reproductive health governance, Accredited Social Health Activist (ASHA) workers are trained and appointed to provide first-contact healthcare at the village level. The ASHA workers promote immunization, make villagers aware about STIs and social determinants of diseases, and primarily, help the villagers obtain reproductive and child health services for prenatal and postnatal care.[19] She reports to the regional Anganwadi center established for India's Integrated Child Development Services (ICDS) to address women and children's malnutrition and hunger and provide wider healthcare services for the villagers. A woman who has previously received a prenatal nutrition package added,

> Generally, the ASHA worker is requested to report pregnancy within the 62nd day to the Anganwadi worker. The Anganwadi worker is then asked to request the government for delivery of 24 eggs, milk, rice, lentils per month

> per pregnant woman until delivery, to ensure maternal and fetal well-being. The produce that I received was good. The government is responsible to ensure the health of the mother. So, the authorities ask local health workers as to why they are not recording pregnancies or spontaneous abortions [within 60 days]. (*Racchabanda, interview,* September 24, 2021)

Srinath Reddy stepped in to fill in about a prior escalation at the District Health Office,

> Actually, before they used to record. The problem is that the [District Health] Officer has a meeting every month. At the time, they did not know that this [high spontaneous abortion rate] is radiation's effect and this is due to UCIL . . . they didn't recognize the problem [to be] so. [DHO] asked [local health workers], "Why you are not monitoring properly, how can the abortion rate be so high in the region? Your record is not proper as a health worker." If the abortion rate was high, they were punished. The Mandal health in-charge was questioned by [the DHO] through a lot of memos. Anganwadi workers said that "these villagers simply say that it is affected by UCIL but there was no conclusion that it was affected by UCIL." (*Racchabanda, interview,* September 24, 2021)

In November 2019, responding to a *Times of India* journalist, U. Sudhakar Reddy, Anganwadi worker J. Vanitamma said, "It is evident there are health problems, but no doctor or scientist could confirm that it is due to uranium contamination."[20] Here, the Anganwadi worker relies on scientific and nuclear expertise to invalidate the attribution made by women and other villagers. Further, both villagers and Srinath Reddy hold that Mandal-level (sub-district) health authorities have advised local health workers to record pregnancies only after 90 days so that district health officials do not question them on reports of increased spontaneous abortions. In such a way, health governance at Tummalapalle is shaped by expert hegemony and attributional claims that circles around the new governance scientific-discursive tool, "maybe." Srinath Reddy states,

> They [health authorities] do not associate reproductive health issues in women to UCIL. That's correct, no one can insist but people are asking, "Why they are not believing [us]?" They did not have evidence [and so] they are not saying the reason and ask the women, "How can you say it is because of UCIL?" They [UCIL] do not say what the level of risk to reproductive health is. The district [health] officials do not have the power to question these lapses [by UCIL] and only state-level authorities [like APPCB] can question. The state-level authorities will intervene only if it is a *serious issue*. At the time, the UCIL will conduct health camps as eyewash but not for reproductive health. (my emphasis, *Racchabanda,* September 24, 2021)

Reproductive illnesses as monitored by decentralized health governance models—through ASHA and Anganwadi workers—are uprooted from their possible environmental contamination origins due to divisible governance. The transcorporeal agential knowledge of the women in Tummalapalle—that because they use more of the contaminated water, absorb irradiated water through their skin, they face more radioactive illnesses—is often contested by public and private doctors. Doctors look for scientific evidence from TUMM's nuclear-industrial complex but it diffuses accountability through new governance techniques of layered/divisible governance, CSR, and "may be [due to natural radiation]." The attributional knowledge of the women about their reproductive illnesses as an effect of radiation exposure is undermined by doctors (Zaretsky 2018; Folkers 2022; Clark 2000). Expert hegemony compounded by gendered roles and radiation's invisibility is further exacerbated by medical advice that follows NRT's imaging of fetuses leading to involuntary childlessness in the region.

During my preliminary visit in September 2021, the first woman I interviewed who had faced an abortion said, "Three months into my first pregnancy, the baby was aborted." As people kept referring to the fetus as a baby, I interrupted the interview and said to Srinath Reddy and my English-speaking translator, "We cannot call it a baby, it's a fetus. What is the word for fetus in Telugu?" Without fully understanding the context of involuntary childlessness in the region, I apathetically reinforced the discourse of pro-choice,[21] fervent in the United States (Laften 2008), on a community facing environmental racism and consequently, involuntary childlessness. Constrained by discourses and topics of interest in the Global North, the theories that emerge from the complex realities of families facing environmental injustice in the Global South barely obtain a representation (Majumdar 2017, 101; Taylor 2008). It took me a while to understand that these communities are facing "stratified reproduction" defined by "power relations in which some categories of people are empowered to nurture and reproduce while others are disempowered" (Rapp and Ginsberg 2007, 1). These relations are shaped extensively by scientific (nuclear and medical) governance and expert hegemony that warrant the final say to UCIL for attributing the cause of contamination.

Medical expertise, informed by diagnosis through NRT, at government and private hospitals determines the reproductive capacities of people at MC Palle and Kottala and undermines their epistemologies of reproduction and reproductive illnesses. The woman continued to speak without paying heed to the conversation about fetus versus baby amongst us: "The baby's growth was not proper. Not completely formed in three months. So, the doctor suggested that it's better to remove it. No actual growth." My translator said, "So, the baby didn't have normal growth." In this conversation, the doctor's diagnosis based on the measurable, graphable fetal images renders the mother's "baby"[22] into medical "baby pictures" that does not conform with biosocial normativity stemming from compulsory able-bodiedness. Rapp (2013) in "real-time fetus" argued that the power of sonographic uterine imaging makes pregnant women identify with fetal images as their babies, making "the pregnancy real from inside" even before the onset of the mother's embodied sensations of kicks and bumps. I asked the woman, "Did the doctor give you a reason [for fetal growth]?"

> Woman: "The doctor asked me, 'In your villages a lot of members face this issue [abortion]. Is there a problem with the water?' I said yes."
>
> Me: "Did you tell the doctor the reason for water contamination?"
>
> Woman: "Doctor advised me to not use the water. If I had asked more questions or told the reason, doctors would have asked, 'Are you the doctor here?'" (everyone laughs; *Racchabanda, interview,* September 24, 2021).

The "problem" of disabled fetal imagery does not emerge *because* of the "natural" formation of the fetus represented by NRT. If the women were to critically analyze the fetal imageries with doctors, they are asked "are you the doctor here?" and this undermines the maternal authority and desires in medical interpretation of fetal imagery. Discounting maternal authority in medical interpretation of the fetal imageries, often recognized as obstetric violence, undermines women's autonomy "to decide freely about their bodies" (Sadler et al. 2016 as cited in Chattopadhyay 2018). In the Global South, Sreeparna Chattopadhyay argues that obstetric violence transcends questions of patient autonomy as it is not useful to "blame" individual providers and institutions that are often under-resourced and overburdened (2022). Instead, she points to the systemic and structural causes of obstetric violence in the Global South, to understand "how different kinds of relational engagements and interventions may lead to different outcomes in terms of the welfare of mothers and infants" (Swartz and Lappeman 2021 as cited in Chattopadhyay 2018). At TUMM, the nuclear-environmental governance by APPCB, UCIL, and AERB, and the health governance by ICDS, Anganwadi center, DHO, Mandal health in-charge, and local private clinics and doctors, forge nuclear-medico-industrial relations that structure institutions of natal care. The nuclear-medico-industrial relations collectively undermine women's embodied knowledge of causation at the environmental level and thereby, the knowledge about radiation's effects.

In the context of Tummalapalle, firstly, medical "advice" reduces reproductive capacity and disability that are "negotiated product[s] of history, power and desires" into a "fact of nature" (Downey and Dumit 1997, 12). Disembedded from maternal desires and knowledge, secondly, "the 'problem' of the disabled" fetus is produced through medical advice that is steeped in notions of "normalcy" (as evoked by my translator) that further constructs disability as undesirable (Davis 2016). In pro-choice debates in the Global North, the real-time fetus in sonograms, disembedded from the mother's embodiment, becomes available for "public viewing and commentary" and operates as a social fetus (Rapp 1997, 38). Whereas, in contaminated places in the Global South like MC Palle, the real-time fetus enters social relations that are "already altered" by chemical relations, alterlife (Murphy 2017). Consequently, maternal autonomy and authority needs to be compulsorily seen in tandem with their embodied knowledge about radioactive contamination. Therefore, in MC Palle, where alterlife is tormented by multiple causes of radioactive contamination with no definitive action, "what disables?" needs to be clearly identified. While the cause of contamination is diffused through the divisible and layered nuclear environmental governance discursive tool, "maybe," the medical response to the effects of contamination on altered and gendered bodies is definite—abortion—as the section below demonstrates. There are no "maybes" in the biomedical relations with the alterlife of the disabled fetal imagery at the nuclear-medico-industrial complex.

The Alterlife of Disabled Fetal Imaginaries

The availability of NRT due to "technological progress" (as expressed in Shiva's words with which I begin the chapter) and doctor's interpretation of the fetal imagery engendering the normate body frame the disability politics of contamination, visibility of radiation, involuntary childlessness, and environmental injustice in the region. For Shiva (a non-resident), the presence of impaired children increases the visibility of radioactive contamination that is otherwise invisible on official registers. Understanding environmental damage through disabled bodies reinforces the double-bind of disability: "the disabled body is necessary to give risk . . . any meaning, and yet [demands that] the disabled body must remain invisible" (Ray 2017; Mannur 2017). However, to analyze the double-bind of disability in the MC Palle villagers, I focus on something else that Shiva said: "Today we have a lot of technologies, they do *scanning* in three months and say there is no leg growth, or another body part has not grown, so abortion." "So, abortion" as medical advice accelerates the state of involuntary childlessness in irradiated MC Palle and Kottala.

Childlessness remains involuntary and complexly intertwined with compulsory able-bodiedness in irradiated MC Palle and Kottala. Abortion of disabled fetuses is less of a matter of individual choice at MC Palle and Kottala.[23] Abortion is a constraint in the "appearance of choice" made in a compulsory able-bodied "system in which there actually is no choice" and is produced by medical expertise, radiation expertise, and lack of top-down governmental intervention, or the new health and environmental governance models (McRuer 2017, 303; Kafer 2013, 162). McRuer also reminds that "the origins of compulsory able-bodiedness" do not emanate from "the rise of industrial capitalism," but understanding about normality is cohered into "a system of compulsory able-bodiedness that similarly emanates from everywhere and nowhere" (2017, 303). As disabled fetal imageries enter the social, biomedical, and nuclear relations that are altered by chemicals, it struggles to go beyond the biomedical imaginary of disabled fetus as undesirable producing a disabled fetal imaginary. In the following section, I locate the multiple locations of power of the compulsory able-bodiedness that shapes involuntary childlessness in the spatiality of environmental contamination at TUMM and not in my English translator's or Shiva's words.

TUMM's Nuclear-Medical-Industrial Complex and the Disabled Fetuses

Monika was part of focus group one that I conducted at the temple located in Mabbuchintalapalle Scheduled Caste[24] (SC) Colony where lower-caste Hindu people are allocated residential plots by the government. People categorized as scheduled and backward castes gathered at the temple and when I tried to ask questions collectively to the group, the women responded, "Every woman's problem is different. You need to ask us one by one before you address us collectively." I agreed and the focus group, initially planned for an hour, went on for about three hours. Every woman had so much to say about menstrual issues and reproductive health concerns including and going beyond pregnancy and childbirth. Towards the end of the final hour, the women became comfortable enough to share about the deeply stigmatized topic of abortion and that was only after Monika opened up to me. Monika said,

> During my periods, I feel a burning sensation around my vagina. I had one [spontaneous] abortion at the start of my third month [of pregnancy]. At Gangi Reddy hospital, they say that it is because of the water in your village, you have these issues. (Focus group 2, October 17, 2021)

My local translator immediately told the group something in Telugu and I noticed that some women laughed, and others sighed. I asked her to translate what she said into Tamil for me to understand. She said, "The daughter of the Gangi Reddy hospital's owner is the wife of Chief Minister Jagan Mohan Reddy. I told her that you could have asked them directly why the water in our village has these issues and why you are having abortions." Although the village is located close to the state's Chief Minister's (CM) hometown which he periodically visits, there is no visibility for the reproductive health issues that "women" face.[25] As the government (under the administration of the CM) does not step in to intervene, the nuclear industry benefits from the uranium reserves in the region and the medical industry benefits from health ailments that *may be* due to the inadequate lining of the tailing pond. The attribution of reproductive health issues to radiation's effect becomes messy in an environment with *may be* natural and anthropogenic radiation exposure. A respondent in the focus group states,

> Every month, women report about their menstrual irregularity (too much white or red) to the health worker. But they advise them to get it checked at town [private] hospital. The women fear that the private hospitals will ask them to operate for even small reproductive health issues and remove the uterus, so they don't go. Also, fearing the cost.

The new environmental governance model in India diffuses the accountability for healthy life onto individual citizens and the private healthcare sector as the public health sector that ensures prenatal, postnatal, and wider reproductive healthcare falls short of its public health goals. Anganwadi workers and Asha workers simultaneously claim, as representatives of public healthcare, that UCIL may not be accountable for the complex reproductive health issues among economically deprived villagers due to the inconclusiveness of the cause of contamination. In private hospitals that benefit the dominant political family, the villagers are advised to carry out expensive surgeries including but not limited to hysterectomy. Bhagyamma[26] and her two daughters-in-law underwent a hysterectomy. She says, "I told my two sons and daughters-in-law to leave the village because I can't afford medical expenses. I had to loan money to get our health checked" (Bhagyamma, *interview,* October 17, 2021). Savitri, whose menstruation lasts up to 60 days and cycles up to 153 days (quite common among many women) stated, "If I get operated and have stitches, I won't be able to work and I am the sole breadwinner of the house . . . " (Focus Group one with women, October 16, 2021*).* Doctors at private hospitals often advise aborting fetuses that do not show "actual" growth. In my second focus group, Saraswati said, "After my first daughter, I conceived but at the seventh month, the doctor told me that the baby is not fully formed and advised me to abort. The doctor told me later, if you want to conceive again and deliver, leave the village." It is not the "availability" and accessibility to "antenatal screening" that invisiblizes radiation and disability as Shiva suggests, but rather "the often-automatic assumption that abortion should follow the discovery of fetal abnormality" (Feldman 2016, 36; Gammeltoft 2007). Savitri stepped in and added, "We do not understand the kind of treatment they give [alluding to the advice for surgeries and abortion].” These words of Savitri call into question whether childlessness is really voluntary in irradiated MC Palle and Kottala.

Reproductive injustice, disability injustice, and environmental injustice come together in the doctor’s interpretation of disabled fetal imageries. Medical advice as informed by NRT imaging, thereby, directly affects lives of disabled fetuses and women altered by chemical relations—their alterlives. However, scholarship in/of India on the social life of NRT is dominated by interest in bourgeois and petit-bourgeois surrogacy desires and struggles (Majumdar 2018; Bharadwaj 2002; Kroløkke 2012) in the management of reproduction that affects economically deprived surrogates. It overlooks the life chances and choices available to economically backward women in contaminated places as their epistemologies of reproductive health/illnesses contests the representations and interpretation of disabled fetal images in NRT. Bound by invisibility and new governance techniques that render the cause of contamination invisible, reproductive health care, although a collective and social issue at MC Palle, is reduced to a matter of individual choice and livelihood chances.

AN ALTERLIFE POSITIONALITY AT THE INTERSECTION OF DISABILITY, ENVIRONMENTAL, AND REPRODUCTIVE JUSTICE

Many villagers are constrained to stay in the village because of lack of resources and these resource constraints, when enabled, generate *an alterlife positionality* that critiques both compulsory able-bodiedness (McRuer 2017) and uncritical mutant optimism (Masco 2004). When I asked Saraswati, “Will you leave if you have the chance, and opportunities to leave the village?” She questioned me, “Why would we stay here with such difficulty if we have the resources and opportunities?” It is the accessibility to healthcare resources that concerns these contaminated communities. The people at MC Palle and Kottala believe that “impairments aren’t disabling, social and architectural barriers are” (Kafer 2013, 8). At the end of the focus group, when I asked the women to state their demands to government, they said:

> We want UCIL to take our land and houses and compensate us for the land. Since agriculture in the area is affected, we do not have a livelihood. If they employ our youth in their industry at least, we will get money and use that money towards our health.” (Focus group 2, October 16, 2021)

People at MC Palle and Kottala recognize that their village is a “world with disability in it” and in their demand for medical insurance, they are simply not deluded by able-bodied futures and temporalities (Garland-Thomson 2017). As "maybe" slows down the responsibility of nuclear experts in addressing the slow environmental violence unfolding at MC Palle and Kottala, "so-abortion" accelerates the choices available for the family through a hegemony of the medical expert. Here, the medical expertise operates with the eugenic logic of "eliminating disability" (Garland-Thomson 2017, 52) instead of relating with disability or in other words, alter-life relationalities. It individualizes reproductive and livelihood choices and fails to enable an alter-governance system in order to provide a collective response to their accessibility concerns in a place altered by chemical relations. The nuclear-medical-industrial complex, "unaltered" by chemical relations, refuses to relate with the disabling conditions at TUMM and thereby, with disability itself. It lacks a relational model of disability even as it remains disabling (Kafer 2013, 6–8).

Nuclear and medical experts operationalize a disembodied science, failing to relate with disability or recognize disability beyond it being "a master trope of human disqualification" (Mitchell and Synder 2000, 3 as quoted in Garland-Thomson 2017, 54). Against eugenic models of disability, disability scholar Rosemarie Garland-Thomson poses a counter-eugenic logic asking, "What do we lose besides the individuals themselves if we eliminate disability and disabled people from the world?" A UCIL employee thankful for the medical insurance benefits he receives, as it helped him treat his child, said,

> Milling and mine operations are safe. My three-year-old has a condition due to genetic issues that the doctors said *probably* runs in the family. UCIL has provided me employment and medical insurance, without which I would have never been able to treat my kid in big hospitals. (Anonymous, *interview*, October 19, 2021)

His response, on the surface, is directly thankful for the medical insurance that supports his disabled child and is rooted in a relational model of disability: that disability is in the built environment rather than in the individual's body. The employee also complexly frames the medical resources as a reward for his contribution to the nuclear-medical-industrial complex. His entitlement to healthy life is measured in terms of his "productivity in capitalist economies" that aids national development that contradicts the basic premise of Garland-Thomson's building a world with disability in it (Garland-Thomson 2017, 54). The eligibility for employment at TUMM that qualifies the villagers for medical insurance is based on a logic of masculine virility: "Men are relatively invulnerable to harm, able to withstand the hazards and risks of the public world, and capable of denying the pains of the human body and the suffering of others . . . [as] the protectors of women, children, and the nation, capable of fighting wars, accepting threats of bodily harm, and shielding others from external risk" (Daniels 2006, 3). At TUMM's nuclear-medical-industrial complex, men who protect "women, children and the nation . . . accepting threat to bodily harm" are provided access to medical resources, making citizenry entitlement to healthy living gendered and "contingent upon the able body" and impeding the building of accessible citizenship (McRuer 2006, 30 as quoted in Minich 2014, 13).

Furthermore, health monitoring in the region is earmarked only for UCIL's employees as a part of its nuclear safety culture. Without UCIL taking accountability for industrial harms, health monitoring does not extend to women and children who may be exposed to low levels of radiation (and wish to know their absorbed doses). UCIL evaded its accountability for irradiation by stating that its operations are safe as it has followed AERB safety guidelines. Without conclusive evidence, the health workers claim that they cannot associate reproductive health of women to radioactive contamination by UCIL, constraining the attention of public health authorities. Nuclear safety thereby shapes whose bodies matter for health surveillance. Nuclear safety practices of occupational surveillance to assess dose equivalent make radiation emerging from nationalist nuclear practices—that is, within milling and mining zones—visible. It invisibilizes the radiation that exists in the environment[27] that "*may be* due to inadequate lining of the tailing pond" to which people other than employees, especially women, are exposed to.

With the medical insurance, the employee's "wounded patriotism" recuperates as it contributes labor towards national nuclear productivity. The recuperation of the wound revitalizes the employee's belief in the scientism of the nuclear safety episteme reproducing attributional relativism—*may be* due to genetics "that runs in the family." Instead of finding a belongingness with the state, the individual finds belonging in the nuclear safety episteme that protects his health (vis-à-vis medical insurance). In an age dominated by the rhetoric "nuclear energy is safe" (Gates 2021), trust in the nuclear safety episteme is paramount to "patriotic body politic," namely, the distrust in the "state for protecting biological health" by its most loyal citizens (Zaretsky 2018, 12).

Reproductive Masculinity and Masculinist State: A Women's Issue?

After focus group one, Shiva came to me and whispered, "Ma'am, it is not only women who face fertility issues. Men too! But nobody talks about it." A local obstetrician-gynecologist confirmed, "Many couples come to the clinic thinking it's a gynecological issue, a problem with women's fertility. But when I send them to fertility clinics, we find out that the problem is with sperm morphology or count. They also, in many instances, happen to be UCIL's employees. But I cannot attribute infertility issues to mine without scientific study proving so" (Local obstetrician-gynecologist, *interview,* October 19, 2021). Men or women do not talk about males' fertility issues because it affects their notion of manhood. Manhood as it shapes compulsory able-bodiedness has significant implications for knowing industrial contamination and the source of health risks. Knowing the contamination, *be*yond the constructs of male virility and compulsory able-bodiedness of men and fetuses, can possibly help in exploring the safeness of operations within plants. As TUMM opines that the uranium concentration in water may *be* natural, health authorities do not associate women's reproductive illnesses to the mining and milling operations (Government of India & Department of Atomic Energy PSU section, 2022). First, the gendered notion that men are not harmed obscures the cause of contamination that may be emergent from mining and milling operations. Second and more significantly, occupational health norms and surveillance that construct male bodies as abled and the socially assumed virility paradoxically obscures the real harm to men's reproductive health that is in need of attention in TUMM, leading to what Cynthia Daniels (2006) calls the paradox of reproductive masculinity.

Health governance as enacted in irradiated zones like around TUMM exhibit some elements of what Cynthia Daniels calls reproductive masculinity (2006, 6–7). The new health governance model at MC Palle and Kottala, as discussed, is situated in India's health governance system with both public and private sectors. The Asha and Anganwadi workers are held accountable for ensuring maternal health and are questioned about the delivery of nutritional packages for pregnant women. Reproductive health care directed towards ensuring prenatal maternal health, although well-intended, marks men as "secondary in biological reproduction" (Daniels 2006). This feeds a belief "men are relatively distant from the health problems of children"' and is based on another element, namely, the belief that they are "less vulnerable to reproductive harms." The latter informs the interest in recruiting men for uranium work and adversely affects health surveillance and healthcare access for women and children lacking abled male bodies' protection as their shields.[28] The TUMM nuclear- industrial complex's desire for male abled bodies in a country where NRT and sonographic imaging are used towards female feticide raises critical questions as much about children assigned female at birth as disabled fetuses (Jha et al. 2006; Majumdar 2018, 100). Are female children favorable to male children who can be employed at UCIL and provide for the transgenerational medical expenses? The logic of nuclear safety thereby is based on what Iris Young calls a masculine protectionist state (2003) and if the women were to question nuclear safety, TUMM's new health, environmental, and nuclear governance model calls their epistemic authority: "[the health workers] ask the women, 'How can you say it is because of UCIL?'" (my emphasis, *Racchabanda, interview,* September 24, 2021).

As families are advised by health workers to go to "town hospitals" due to a failed public health care system, families approach the fertility problem with the mindset that "men are relatively distant from the health problems of children" (Daniels 2006). In MC Palle's biosocial registers of becoming irradiated, radiation exposure is made visible through the encounter with irradiated water in the borewell and so, as Anjali remarked, women are imagined to be more exposed and the reproductive health issues are associated with their bodies. Even as couples try to diagnose their reproductive health issues, the first stop becomes a gynecologist's clinic. A line is clearly drawn between exposures to women and men, the former arising from increased exposure to irradiated water that *may be* natural/anthropogenic as against the exposure to the latter who work in mines—because as the employee who had the medical insurance to treat his kid remarked "milling and mine operations are safe." Ultimately, the health and life chances of women, disabled fetuses, and men remain exposed to risks in the scientific contestation over evidential attribution of contamination.

As accountability remains diffused by new governance models for addressing nuclear, environmental, and health risks, "the ideological blueprint" of TUMM's nuclear-medical-industrial complex becomes visible: extraction based on layered/divisible governance, nuclear and medical expert hegemony, inaccessible citizenship for women, masculine protectionism and paradoxes of masculine reproductivity that I have demonstrated until now through the "theoretical power of" disabled fetal imagery (Siebers 2010, 105 as quoted in Minich 2004, 6). When reminding about the theoretical power of disabled bodies, Siebers also reminds us that disabled people hold "little power in the social world" (Siebers 2010, 105 as quoted in Minich 2004, 6). TUMM's nuclear-medical-industrial complex that shapes radiation's visibility through disability while keeping disability itself invisible through able-bodied masculine productivity—or simply, the double-bind of disability embedded in TUMM's nuclear-medical-industrial complex—denotes the state's failure of relating with disability. In this frame, individuals are disciplined to pull themselves up by their bootstraps and make "choices" (the only available one) that advances nuclear productivity of the state in order to [be able to] protect one's own "biological health." As the state's role to protect "biological health" dissipates and the protection of health as a matter of individual choices and "free market" accrues, the new nuclear, medical, and environmental governance models emerge at the horizon of a self-reliant nuclear nation that India aspires to be (Zaretsky 2018).

CONCLUSION

The attributional relativism achieved through the new governance material-semiotic tool "may be" sustains these new governance models. The nuclear safety episteme that a safely designed tailing pond, monitoring borewells, and safety emission standards will effectively protect people from irradiation was employed to avert accountability and sustain attributional relativism. As the role to protect people from irradiation shifted from government to safe technologies and corporate employment benefits, TUMM's nuclear-medical-industrial complex was born. Doctors and people involved in this complex resorted to individual choices, namely abortion and forced displacement to address and respond to lives altered by irradiation. An individual can, however, choose only when acting within the logical framework of a masculine protectionist state: masculine reproductivity, women's epistemic invisibility, scientific and medical expert hegemony, and eugenic logic of disability. The nuclear safety episteme thereby creates a new nuclear bureaucracy which privileges the free market (as in, health services are available for those who have medical insurance) and individual choices over the state role in "protection of biological health" (Zaretsky 2008).

Furthermore, the new nuclear bureaucracy driven by nuclear industrial aspirations recognizes "the ferruginous hawk, the pygmy rabbit, and the larkspur" in contaminated nuclear sites (Masco 2004 533). This, according to nuclear scholar Joseph Masco, is redefining "the division between normal, abnormal, and pathological," as "contaminated nature is recognized to be not only valuable and robust but, to greater or lesser degrees, ever present." A mutant honeybee (Masco 2004, 536) or irradiated fruit flies (Cram 2016) serve a different purpose—as they complicate radioactive containment, the nuclear state accepts radiation as "ever present" and "porous." Radioporosity—that is, a recognition that radiation is always already porous, busting myths of its containment—is often asserted by the state and the industry only when it suits nuclear profit calculations (Shaik Ali 2022; 2023). However, maybe irradiated women, men, and fetuses in MC Palle and Kottala remind that the presence of mutant ecologies does not always translate into reinvention of what is normal, abnormal, and pathological. When the nuclear state stares at the human body (and its "integrity") for nuclear productivity, masculine reproductivity, and through the eugenic logic of disability, mutant optimism is shunned, the normate body is upheld, and the abnormal becomes pathological and in need of elimination.

The ethnographic enthusiasm for new ecologies of irradiated zones necessarily has to address how the state relates with normate bodies and disability by fully taking into account its nuclear calculations, productive bodies, and the profits accruing thereof. Whereas in places where "radiation" is recognized as ever present and mutant ecologies are seen as new lifeforms like Chernobyl (Zimmer 2022) and Hanford (Cram 2016), the division between normal and abnormal continues to shape the nuclear-medical-industrial complex's approach to disability around TUMM that denies its role in radiation contamination. Even as farmers and women explore how to live on damaged land, generating possibilities from damage (Murphy 2017), and do not call for shutting down TUMM's extractive capitalism, their alterlife positionality emphasizes the "pain" of being on damaged land as an exercise of relating with disability (Kafer 2013, 6). A couple thankful for medical insurance for treating their unhealthy child, a farmer trying to grow food on severely damaged land, and women asserting their knowledge of radioactive contamination as much as they enable damage and its possibilities highlight the pain of extraction. Because prolonged exposure to irradiated water kills crops, Ramanjenellu has to drive up to his farm every hour during daylight to unlimitedly water his plants. Whereas before contamination he drove up to his farm once in the morning to leave the water on and again in the evening to switch it off. Farmers Ram Mohan and Vinod said, "Now all the villages around us know that there are a lot of childbearing issues in our village. We find it difficult to get our youth married" (Vinod family, *interview,* October 22, 2021). As Feldman remarks, "Part of the desire of the infertile for children is that they live in real societies where involuntary childlessness may affect their lives in very tangible and harmful ways. So, the needs of the infertile become an important starting point in thinking about the technologies and their implications" (1987, 24). These anecdotes point to the pain of becoming irradiated as they relate with disability and damage for, sometimes, productive capacities and, at rare times, generative possibilities (Murphy 2017, 10).

In the age of Anthropocene, a new nuclear environmental-health bureaucracy, and new medical technologies, an alterlife positionality, taken anywhere (in governance, academic, and popular culture), attends to possibilities of damage with a critical approach to mutant optimism that relates with the pain emerging from scientific hegemony and environmental violence—emergent in the ways these triadic spatio-temporal forces relate with disability.

NOTES

1. Michelle Murphy lays out (both injurious and political) kinship as a significant political dimension of alter-life. They also simultaneously claim that responsibility in a world that is already altered by chemical relations needs to go beyond building alter-relations, to "dismantle violent infrastructures" (Murphy 2017, 11). In this way,

people's adaptation to environmental violence that engenders alter-life is never a justification for further environmental violence.

2. *Racchabanda* are elevated platforms below a tree where villagers meet to discuss; it's a village meeting. Most of my ethnographic interviews carried out in public places in India can barely be controlled to be one-on-one. People drop in and drop out, sign consent forms, and add their two cents.

3. For satellite images showing the picture of the area, see Puzhakkal (2019).

4. Bananas are the main crop in the area. Between the fiscal years 2015–2016 and 2019–2020, the number of villages planned for banana cultivation decreased from 18 (of 136 villages) to 12 (of 53 villages) in YSR district.

5. Calculated at an exchange rate, USD 1 = INR 80 in the article.

6. Although the edited volume concerns medical technologies and places health-related concerns at the center of analysis, this chapter is framed around the primary matter of concern for the villagers—nuclear environmental-health contamination and regulation of it. I first analyze the environmental contamination and secondly, elaborate on the health aspects yielding an account of nuclear environmental health.

7. If the problem was in the USA and involved the EPA, as I have noticed works in the Global North, I would not have to explain the constitution of these authorities but since the readers in the West are not familiar with the regulatory constitution in India, I do so.

8. APPCB spent around INR 51 lakhs (or USD 63, 750) on scientific analysis of the cost of contamination carried over by Indian Institute of Technology, Madras. See "Issues at Operating Uranium Mines and Mills—India." n.d. https://www.wise-uranium.org/umopin.html.

9. Layered governance is governance through risk fragmentation and it often precedes "divisible governance." STS scholars Timothy Naele and Kristy Howey (2022) define divisible governance as the "fragmentation of environmental risks between temporal and jurisdictional categories, allowing interested state and nonstate actors to superficially appear to protect the environment while actually deferring, forestalling, or eliminating their accountability for the consequences" (5).

10. Nuclear safety and radiation protection may sound like they are the same but were historically different categories and were made one and the same through a history of standard setting (Creager 2015; Boudia 2007, 2014; Walker 2000). For the methodological use of the differentiation between these two categories in STS-ethnographic research, see Shaik Ali (2022). I refuse to regard regulation by nuclear safety as radiation protection although the International Atomic Energy Agency has made it one and the same through a history of standard setting. Read *Fundamental Safety Principles* (European Atomic Energy Community et. al 2006).

11. I primarily regard nuclear safety as a phenomenotechnique, a regulatory technique that doesn't represent the reality that nuclear energy is safe but rather shapes a world where nuclear energy is constructed to be safe. Through its very scientific organization, nuclear safety as a knowledge framework lays the possibility for thinking about nuclear regulation, impeding scientific curiosity to explore other epistemologies of nuclear regulation (Bachelard 2002).

12. Similar response has been given for contamination around another uranium mine and mill in Jadugoda, Jharkhand State (National Green Tribunal 2022).

13. Initially, when I had visited villages and TUMM, my primary research interest was to build a sensory archive of radiation in India as a project of the Critical Nuclear Studies I was framing in my dissertation. Through well-organized sensory and multispecies ethnographic research, I looked for the ways human and nonhuman, *as bodies that know or epistemic bodies*, sensed the invisible "radiation" and complexly perceptible "radioactive contamination." More than how radiation affected people,'s lives and victimized them, I was interested in understanding how people perceived radiation and attributed health and environmental contamination to the nuclear facility as emplaced knowers (Pink 2015).

14. On the biomedical burden of ionizing and non-ionizing radiation, see Kaur (2020) and Mukherjee (2020).

15. Anjali is a college-going student and claims that her menstrual cramps, skin itching, and pigmentation is reduced when she lives in her college hostel, around 20 km from her native village MC Palle.

16. India's nuclear program is imagined to be completed in three stages where its nuclear fuel dependency would shift from uranium sourced from abroad to thorium that is mined and milled within the territories of India, or indigenous radioactive material. India has one-third of the world's thorium resources. The postcolonial country, marred by the fear of recolonization, in the 1950s adopted this plan to make India into a "self-reliant" nation. Since 40 percent of India's uranium inventory is indigenously mined and milled at TUMM, TUMM is framed to make India into a self-reliant and developed nation (Asani 2018).

17. To the villagers' contamination reports, UCIL states that since it has followed the safety guidelines provided by the AERB, its operations do not contaminate. This belief is embedded in the nuclear safety episteme discussed in the first section.

18. On compounded vulnerability, see Versey (2021).

19. ASHA workers do not receive a government salary but are provided fixed payment and monetary incentives for every routine reproductive health service. For every successful delivery, ASHA workers in rural areas earn INR 300.

20. See also, Reddy (2019).

21. As Majumdar (2017) explains, "Abortion has never occupied a pro-choice and pro-life debate in India, again largely due to the population policies of the state that have encouraged family planning" (101).

22. Disclaimer: I am pro-choice.

23. On the dysgenic state, disability, and environmental racism, see Bridges (2022).

24. The use of lower-caste bodies in the mine to carry out work in radiation fields is institutionally streamlined at TUMM, obscuring the caste politics that underlies it. It has direct implications for social and environmental injustice and is deeply sedimented by the scientific belief in the nuclear safety episteme. To read more, see Shaik Ali 2022. Although it is significant health and environmental injustice, I will not be able to address it within the scope and length of this chapter on new health governance and fetal imageries (and to be generous to the readers).

25. From secondary data, door-to-door survey, and interviews, 44 percent of pregnancies ended in spontaneous abortions between January and July 2021 as against a universal average of 30 percent of pregnancies (Pallikadavath and Stones 2005).

26. Bhagyamma is an agricultural laborer and does agriculture on a loaned one-acre of land. She saved up money in small amounts and built one of the biggest houses in the middle of MC Palle village for her two daughters-in-law, sons, their children, and herself to stay in. But because of the health effects on reproduction, she asked them to leave the village. She says, "I wanted to see my grandchildren in the house. Now, every day, I return from the farm and there is no one in the house. I live in such a big haunted house."

27. In September 2021, due to heavy rains, the radioactive material in the tailing pond was washed off into nearby agricultural land and villages. Since radioactive levels of the tailings are generally within the safety limit of 6–8 ppb, the authorities told villagers that there is nothing to worry about (Express News Service 2021), whereas a low level of radiation is said to affect women and children adversely (Folkers 2022).

28. Effect of radiation on sperm has remained contested and unfinished, helping both anti- and pro-nuclear stakeholders to use scientific studies that further their cause (Daniels 2006, 123–24).

REFERENCES

Abraham, Itty. 2012. "Geopolitics and Biopolitics in India's High Natural Background Radiation Zone." *Science, Technology and Society* 17 (1): 105–22.

APPCB (Andhra Pradesh Pollution Control Board). 2007. *Consent for Establishment Order.* No. 103/PCB/CFE/RO-TPT/HO/2007–86. Kurnool, AP: APPCB, March 5. Srinath Reddy Personal Archives, Pulivendula, AP.

———. 2018. *UCIL's Responses to Show-cause Notice and APPCB's observations.* Lr. No. 90/APPCB/ZO/KNL/2018." Kurnool, AP: APPCB, April 19. Srinath Reddy Personal Archives, Pulivendula, AP.

———. 2019. *UCIL's Responses to Show-Cause Notice*. Kurnool, AP: APPCB, August [8–14?]. Manuscript. Srinath Reddy Personal Archives, Pulivendula, AP.

Asani, C.K. 2018. "Development of Alkali Leaching Technology: Key to Self Sufficiency in Uranium Production in India." Paper presented at *Uranium Raw Material for the Nuclear Fuel Cycle: Exploration, Mining, Production, Supply and Demand, Economics and Environmental Issues (Uram-2018): An International Symposium Organized by the International Atomic Energy Agency in Cooperation with the OECD Nuclear Energy Agency and the World Nuclear Association and Held in Vienna, 25–29 June 2018*. IAEA. https://conferences.iaea.org/event/146/contributions/5225/contribution.pdf.

Bharadwaj, Aditya. 2002. "Conception Politics: Medical Egos, Media Spotlights, and the Contest over Test-Tube Firsts in India." In *Infertility around the Globe: New Thinking on Childlessness, Gender, and Reproductive Technologies*, edited by Marcia Claire Inhorn and Frank van Balen, 315–34. Berkeley: University of California Press.

Boudia, Soraya. 2014. "From Threshold to Risk: Exposure to Low Doses of Radiation and Its Effects on Toxicants Regulation." In *Toxicants, Health and Regulation since 1945*, edited by Soraya Boudia and Nathalie Jas, 71–88. London, England: Pickering & Chatto.

———. 2007. "Global Regulation: Controlling and Accepting Radioactivity Risks," *History & Technology* 23 (4): 389–406.

Boudia, Soraya, Angela N.H. Creager, Scott Frickel, Emmanuel Henry, Nathalie Jas, Carsten Reinhardt, and Jody A. Roberts. 2018. "Residues: Rethinking Chemical Environments." *Engaging Science, Technology, and Society* 4: 165–78.

Bridges, Khiara M. 2022. "The Dysgenic State: Environmental Injustice and Disability-Selective Abortion Bans." *California Law Review* 110 (2): 297–369.

Burch, Karly Ann. 2019. "When Overflow Is the Rule: The Evolution of the Transnational Nuclear Assemblage and Its Technopolitical Tools for Framing Human–Radionuclide Relationality." *Geoforum* 107 (December): 66–76. https://doi.org/10.1016/j.geoforum.2019.10.011.

Chattopadhyay, Sreeparna. 2022. "Individuals, institutions, and the global political economy: Unpacking intentionality in obstetric violence." In *Birth Controlled: Selective Reproduction and Neo-Liberal Eugenics in South Africa and India,* edited by Amrita Pande. England: Manchester University Press.

Clark, Claudia. 2000. *Radium Girls, Women and Industrial Health Reform: 1910–1935*. The University of North Carolina Press.

Conley, John M., and Cynthia A. Williams. 2017. "Engage, Embed, and Embellish: Theory versus Practice in the Corporate Social Responsibility Movement." *Human Rights and Corporations*, March, 445–82. https://doi.org/10.4324/9781315252964-12.

Cram, Shannon. 2016. "Wild and Scenic Wasteland: Conservation Politics in the Nuclear Wilderness." *Environmental Humanities* 7 (1): 89–105.

Creager, Angela N.H. 2018. "Human Bodies as Chemical Sensors: A History of Biomonitoring for Environmental Health and Regulation." *Studies in History and Philosophy of Science* Part A 70: 70–81.

———. 2014. "Radiation, cancer, and mutation in the atomic age." *Historical Studies in the Natural Sciences* 45 (1): 14–48.

Daniels, Cynthia R. 2006. *Exposing Men: The Science and Politics of Male Reproduction.* Oxford, England: Oxford University Press.

Davis, Lennard J. 2016. *Enforcing Normalcy: Disability, Deafness, and the Body.* New York: Verso Books.

Downey, Gary Lee, and Joseph Dumit. 1997. *Cyborgs & Citadels: Anthropological Interventions in Emerging Sciences and Technologies*. Santa Fe, NM: School of American Research Press.

European Atomic Energy Community, the Food and Agriculture Organization of the United Nations, the International Labour Organization, the International Maritime Organization, the OECD Nuclear Energy Agency, the Pan American Health Organization, the United 321 Nations Environment Programme and the World Health Organization. 2006. *Fundamental Safety Principles: Safety Fundamentals.* Vienna: IAEA.

Express News Service. 2021. “No overflow from UCIL pond, clarifies Atomic Energy Regulatory Board.” *The New Indian Express*, September 12, 2021. Accessed December 29, 2022. https://www.newindianexpress.com/states/andhra-pradesh/2021/sep/12/no-over flow-from-ucil-pond-clarifies-atomic-energy-regulatory-board-2357547.html.

Feldman, R. 1987. “The politics of the new reproductive technologies.” *Critical Social Policy* 7 (19): 21–39. https://doi.org/10.1177/026101838700701902.

Folkers, Cynthia. 2022. “Disproportionate Impacts of Radiation Exposure on Women, Children, and Pregnancy: Taking Back Our Narrative.” In *Connecting to the Living History of Radiation Exposure*, edited by Jacob Hamblin and Linda M. Richards, 31–66. Cham: Springer Nature Switzerland. https://doi.org/10.1007/978-3-031-18758-2_3.

Gammeltoft, Tine M. 2007. “Prenatal Diagnosis in Postwar Vietnam: Power, Subjectivity, and Citizenship.” *American Anthropologist* 109(1): 153–63. http://www.jstor.org/stable/4496594.

Garland-Thomson, Rosemarie. 2017. “Building a World with Disability in It.” In *Culture—Theory—Disability: Encounters between Disability Studies and Culture Studies*, edited by Anne Waldschmidt, Hanjo Berressem, and Moritz Ingwersen, 51–62. Bielefeld: Verlag transcript.

———. 1996. *Extraordinary Bodies: Figuring Physical Disability in American Culture and Literature*. New York: Columbia University Press.

Gates, Bill. 2021. *How to Avoid a Climate Disaster: The Solutions We Have and the Breakthroughs We Need.* London: Penguin Random House.

Government of India & Department of Atomic Energy PSU section. 2022. *DAE's comments on News Item Published in the Telugu Newspaper Named “Eenadu Andhra Pradesh Edition” dated August 7th 2021 entitled “Do Pollution Leaks Apply to Uranium? In Kadapa District, Andhra Pradesh.* Shekhar C. Chavan. No. 10/12(3)/2022/PSU/9556. Mumbai: Department of Atomic Energy. Online Database. Accessed January 3, 2022. https://greentribunal.gov.in/sites/default/files/news_updates/COMMENTS-OPINION%20BY%20DEPARTMENT%20OF%20ATOMIC%20ENERGY%20IN%20OA%20 NO.%20245%20of%202022%20(In%20re%20%20News%20item%20published%20in%20the%20Telugu%20Newspaper%20named,%20Eenadu,%20 . . .).pdf.

Hatakeyama, Sumiko. 2022. “Let Chromosomes Speak: The Cytogenetics Project at the Atomic Bomb Casualty Commission (ABCC).” In *Connecting to the Living History of Radiation Exposure*, edited by Jacob Hamblin and Linda M. Richards, 107–26. Cham: Springer Nature Switzerland. https://doi.org/10.1007/978-3-031-18758-2_6.

Hecht, Gabrielle. 2012. *Being Nuclear: Africans and the Global Uranium Trade.* Cambridge, MA: The MIT Press.

Howey, Kirsty, and Timothy Neale. 2022. “Divisible Governance: Making Gas-Fired Futures during Climate Collapse in Northern Australia.” *Science, Technology & Human Values* 20 (10): 1–30.

IAEA (International Atomic Energy Agency). 2007. *IAEA Safety Glossary: Terminology Used in Nuclear Safety and Radiation Protection.* Vienna: IAEA.

Jha, P., R. Kumar, P. Vasa, N. Dhingra, D. Thiruchelvam, and R. Moineddin. 2006. "Low Male-to-Female Sex Ratio of Children Born in India: National Survey of 1.1 Million Households." *The Lancet* 367: 211–18.

Kafer, Alison. 2013. *Feminist, Queer, Crip*. Bloomington: Indiana University Press.

Kaur, Raminder. 2020. *Kudankulam: The Story of an Indo-Russian Nuclear Power Plant.* New Delhi: Oxford University Press.

Kimura, Aya H. 2016. *Radiation Brain Moms and Citizen Scientists: The Gender Politics of Food Contamination after Fukushima.* London: Duke University Press.

Kriksey, Eben. 2020. *The Mutant Project: Inside the Global Race to Genetically Modify Humans.* New York: St. Martin's Press.

Kroløkke, Charlotte. 2012. "From India with Love: Troublesome Citizens of Fertility Travel." *Cultural Politics* 8 (2): 307–25.

Laflen, Angela. 2008. "(Re)presenting the fetus: the limits of objective vision in 'Birthmates' and 'The Ultrasound.'" *Mosaic: A Journal for the Interdisciplinary Study of Literature* 41 (4): 111+. *Gale Literature Resource Center* (accessed February 4, 2023). https://link.gale.com/apps/doc/A191218013/LitRC?u=anon~5d218c55&sid=googleScholar&xid=b3ac32c5.

Majumdar, Anindita. 2017. *Transnational Commercial Surrogacy and the (Un)Making of Kin in India*. Delhi: Oxford University Press.

Mannur, Anita. 2017. "'That Night': Seeing Bhopal Through the Lens of Disability and Environmental Justice Studies." In *Disability Studies and the Environmental Humanities: Toward an Eco-Crip Theory*, 381–402. University of Nebraska Press.

Masco, Joseph. 2004. "Mutant Ecologies: Radioactive Life in Post–Cold War New Mexico." *Cultural Anthropology* 19 (4): 517–50.

McRuer, Robert. 2017. "Compulsory Able-Bodiedness and Queer/Disabled Existence." Essay. In *The Disability Studies Reader*, edited by Lennard J. Davis, 88–99. New York: Routledge.

Minich, Julie Avril. 2014. *Accessible Citizenships Disability, Nation, and the Cultural Politics of Greater Mexico*. Philadelphia, PA: Temple University Press.

Mitchell, David T. and Sharon L. Snyder. 2000. *Narrative Prosthesis: Disability and the Dependencies of Discourse*. Ann Arbor: The University of Michigan Press.

Mitchell, M. X. 2022. "The Cosmology of Evidence: Suffering, Science, and Biological Witness After Three Mile Island." In *Connecting to the Living History of Radiation Exposure*, edited by Jacob Hamblin and Linda M. Richards, 7–29. Cham: Springer Nature Switzerland. https://doi.org/10.1007/978-3-031-18758-2_2.

Mukherjee, Rahul. 2020. *Radiant Infrastructures: Media, Environment, and Cultures of Uncertainty.* London: Duke University Press.

Murphy, Michelle. 2017. "What Can't a Body Do," *Catalyst* 3 (1): 1–15.

National Green Tribunal. 2022. Reply/Opinion of Uranium Corporation of India Ltd., (Respondent No.9). M.V. Suresh. No. 245 of 2022. New Delhi: National Green Tribunal. Online Database. Accessed March 15, 2023. https://greentribunal.gov.in/sites/default/files/news_updates/REPLY-OPINION%20BY%20URANIUM%20CORP.%20OF%20INDIA%20LTD%20(UCIL)%20IN%20OA%20NO.%20245%20OF%202022%20(item%20published%20in%20the%20Telugu

%20Newspaper%20named,%20Eenadu,%20Andhra%20Pradesh%20edition%20 . . .).pdf

Pallikadavath, Saseendran and R. William Stones. 2005. "Miscarriage in India: A Population-Based Study." *Fertility and Sterility* 84 (2): 516–18.

Petryna, Adrianna. 2013. *Life Exposed: Biological Citizenship after Chernobyl*. Princeton, NJ: Princeton University Press.

Pranesh, S.R. 2018. "Letter to the Joint Chief Environmental Engineer." Manuscript. Srinath Reddy Personal Archives, Pulivendula, Andhra Pradesh.

Puzhakkal, Dheeshma. 2019. "A View from the Satellite: Kadapa Turns into a Uranium Cemetery." *Newsmeter*, November 25, 2019. https://m.newsmeter.in/article/a-view-from-the-satellite-kadapa-turns-into-a-uranium-cemetery-and-the-people-are-its/a-view-from-the-satellite-kadapa-turns-into-a-uranium-cemetery-and-the-people-are-its-victims.

Rapp, Rayna. 2000. *Testing Women, Testing the Fetus: The Social Impact of Amniocentesis in America*. New York: Routledge.

———. 1997. "Real Time Fetus: The Role of the Sonogram in the Age of Monitored Reproduction." Essay. In *Cyborgs & Citadels: Anthropological Interventions in Emerging Sciences and Technologies*, edited by Gary Lee Downey and Joseph Dumit, 31–48. Santa Fe, NM: School of American Research Press.

Rapp, Rayna, and Faye Ginsburg. 2009. "Enlarging Reproduction, Screening Disability." Essay. In *Reproductive Disruptions Gender, Technology, and Biopolitics in the New Millennium*, edited by Marcia C. Inhorn, 1–34. New York: Berghahn Books. https://www.researchgate.net/publication/265311568_Enlarging_Reproduction_Screening_Disability.

Ray, Sarah Jaquette. 2017. "Risking Bodies in the Wild: The 'Corporeal Unconscious' of American Adventure Culture." In *Disability Studies and the Environmental Humanities: Toward an Eco-Crip Theory*, edited by Sarah Jacquette Ray and Jay Sibara, 29–73. Lincoln: University of Nebraska Press.

Reddy, Sudhakar U. 2019. "Health Scare in Villages near UCIL's Tailing Pond in Kadapa." *The Times of India*, November 15. Accessed Jan 15, 2023. https://timesofindia.indiatimes.com/city/hyderabad/health-scare-in-villages-near-ucils-tailing-pond-in-kadapa/articleshow/72062274.cms

Rennie, Richard. 2005. "The Historical Origins of an Industrial Disaster: Occupational Health and Labour Relations at the Fluorspar Mines, St. Lawrence, Newfoundland, 1933–1945." *Labour / Le Travail* 55 (January): 107–42.

Salter, Cynthia L., Abisola Olaniyan, Dara D. Mendez, and Judy C. Chang. 2021. "Naming Silence and Inadequate Obstetric Care as Obstetric Violence is a Necessary Step for Change." *Violence Against Women* 27 (8): 1019–27.

Shaik Ali, Misria. 2023. "Experiments on Radioporosity: A Response to Decaying Trust at YSR District, Andhra Pradesh." *Centre for 21st Century Studies* (forthcoming).

———. 2022. "Becoming Irradiated: The Epistemic Politics of Neglect along India's Nuclear Fuel Cycle." PhD Dissertation, New York: Rensselaer Polytechnic Institute.

Shiva, Vandana. 1988. *Staying Alive: Women, Ecology, and Development*. Berkeley, CA: North Atlantic Books.

Sikina, Maia. 2022. "Resistance and Resilience in Uranium Mines in Jharkhand." In *People Against Nuclear Energy: Anti-Nuclear Movements in India,* edited by Ajmal Khan, 163–89. New Delhi: Safe Publications and Yodapress.

Sklyar, Alekandr. 2019. "Living in Post-Fukushima Grey Zones: Family Decisions in the Wake of Nuclear Disaster." PhD Dissertation, Ann Arbor: University of Michigan.

Swartz, Leslie, and Maura Lappeman. 2021. "Making Care Better in the Context of Violence: The Limits of Blame." *Violence Against Women* 27 (8): 1028–34.

Taylor, Janelle S. 2008. *The Public Life of the Fetal Sonogram Technology, Consumption, and the Politics of Reproduction.* New Brunswick, NJ: Rutgers University Press.

UCIL (Uranium Corporation of India Limited) and Mecon Ltd. 2020. Environmental Impact Assessment Report for Expansion of Tummalapalle Uranium Project from 9.0 to 13.5 Lakh TPA in YSR (Kadapa) District, AP. Kurnool, AP: APPCB. https://pcb.ap.gov.in/APPCBDOCS/Tenders_Noti//EIA-EMP-Tummalapalle_compressed-301-750-1-200.pdf

Ureta, Sebastian. 2020. "Ruination Science: Producing Knowledge from a Toxic World." *Science, Technology, & Human Values* 46 (1): 29–52.

Versey, Shellae. 2021. "Missing Pieces in the Discussion on Climate Change and Risk: Intersectionality and Compounded Vulnerability." *Behavioral and Brain Sciences* 8 (1): 67–75. https://journals.sagepub.com/doi/pdf/10.1177/2372732220982628

Walker, J. Samuel. 2000. *Permissible Dose: A History of Radiation Protection in the Twentieth Century.* Berkeley: University of California Press.

Wellock, Thomas Raymond. 2021. *Safe Enough? A History of Nuclear Power and Accident Risk.* Oakland, CA: University of California Press.

Young, Iris Marion. 2003. "The Logic of Masculinist Protection: Reflections on the Current Security State." *Signs* 29 (1): 1–25.

Zaretsky, Natasha. 2018. *Radiation Nation: Three Mile Island and the Political Transformation of the 1970s.* New York: Columbia University Press.

Zimmer, Katarina. 2022. "Scientists Can't Agree about Chernobyl's Impact on Wildlife." *Knowledgable Magazine*, July 2, 2022.

Chapter 5

Menstrual Futures

Medical Technologies' Impact on Beliefs about "Normal" Bleeding

Amber Nicole Brooks

Since the 1946 animated Disney film *The Story of Menstruation*, to the 2022 Disney movie *Turning Red*, adolescent milestones, namely menarche or the onset of menstruation, have been a thread of discourse within popular culture in the United States. Since the late nineteenth century, medical discourse on menstruation has been at times contentious with myriad perspectives and theories: for example, higher education harms women's reproductive system, women must rest while menstruating, menstruation is pathological, menstruation is normal and necessary, menstruation is an unnecessary burden, menstrual suppression is dangerous, menstrual suppression is healthy, and so on. A 2020 article in *The Atlantic*, titled "No One Has to Get Their Period Anymore: Menstruating is Painful, Expensive, and . . . Unnecessary?" solidifies menstrual suppression as a topic of discourse in the public imagination (Renault). For a lay audience, Renault explains that most doctors today agree there is no medical necessity for periods, and doctors prescribe amenorrhea to relieve symptoms of various conditions. "We now have the technology to make periods optional," explains Dr. Sophia Yen from Stanford Medical School (qtd. in Renault). The technology Yen refers to includes birth control pills and intrauterine devices (IUDs).

Scholars have produced research on birth control pills, including pills approved and marketed specifically for menstrual suppression: for example, Seasonale (released 2003) and Lybrel (released 2007). In addition to the pill, some hormonal IUDs are also menstrual suppression technologies. In this chapter, I will examine menstrual suppression technologies' impact on changing beliefs about menstruation in the United States. First, I will provide a brief look at historical perspectives on menstruation. Second, I will outline key processes of biomedicalization and Feminist STS perspectives that consider how medical technologies change social relations, institutions, and beliefs about what is normal. Third, I will examine existing critical scholarship on menstrual suppression from a sociological and STS perspective. Fourth, I will discuss evolving menstrual scripts and examine discourses around the Mirena and Kyleena IUDs, analyzing how new menstrual scripts demonstrate and construct new definitions around menstrual bleeding, and how these discourses produce new subjectivities. Lastly, I will outline possible research paths for exploring menstrual futures.

Based on this analysis, I argue that although birth control pills marketed for menstrual suppression have already initiated the normalization of eliminating periods, the Mirena and Kyleena IUD marketing materials further normalize lessening or eliminating menstruation by flexibly defining HMB (heavy menstrual bleeding) as a medical condition that demands treatment. Additionally, by producing a gendered subjectivity of responsibilization and agency, these discourses encourage reflexive self-surveillance and optimization of the body, illustrating the biopolitical script that Takeshita (2012) terms the practice of self. More broadly, some of the materials illustrate a near lifetime of menses, which is an expansion of biomedicalization.

HISTORICAL PERSPECTIVES ON MENSTRUATION

In 1874, Edward H. Clarke popularized the theory of menstrual disability, claiming that women cannot both go through puberty and be educated as men are; they need rest due to a limited energy supply, and mental or brain work can cause long-term harm to reproductive capacity and so-called maternal instincts (Bullough and Voght 1973; Martin 1987; 2001). In the late nineteenth century, several scholars published widely about the dangers of mental work and higher education for girls and women who menstruate, arguing that the mental work draws resources away from the reproductive system, risking long-term harm (Kellogg 1882; Clouston 1883; Maudsley 1884). These arguments appeared in medical books and medical journals, as well as a series for the public in *Popular Science Monthly* from 1883–1884 titled "Female Education from a Medical Point of View" (Clouston 1883–84). However, this perspective did not escape critique and rebuttal. Bullough and Voght (1973) explain how Annie G. Howes et al. published the first empirical research around the issue in 1885, entitled "Health Science Statistics of Women College Graduates: Report of Special Committee of the Association of College Alumnae," which reported no significant differences in health for college women. One year later, John Dewey published a rebuttal to Clouston in *Popular Science Monthly*, arguing that studying wasn't harmful to women's reproductive system and that stress related to personal matters was most harmful; Dewey's argument drew on statistical evidence within the Massachusetts Labor Bureau report on the health of American college women (Dewey 1886; Bullough and Voght 1973). It's important to recognize that these arguments and discourse are focused on white privileged women, who have access to college and whose reproductive vitality is of concern to these scholars.

Brumberg (1993) argues that the "sanitary products industry was implicated in the long-term transformation of menarche from a maturation event to a hygienic crisis" (127). From 1890 to WWII, many girls learned about menstruation through reading informational books on health and hygiene. Lister's antisepsis and germ theory informed a cultural shift to menstrual management (napkins, rags, linens), where pads were seen as a source of disease and taboo menstrual blood was considered dangerous. Hygiene and washing were emphasized. In 1913, the American Medical Association (AMA) published *Daughter, Mother, Father: A Story for Girls*. After the war, the social hygiene movement incorporated menstrual preparedness into schools and programs such as the Girl Scouts, as part of broader Progressive Era curricula. The 1920s brought Kotex advertisements focused on hygiene, targeting college and working women. The 1960s advertisements targeted younger adolescents and the broader adolescent experience, focusing more on convenience (and avoiding embarrassment) rather than hygiene, marking a shift to commercialization (Brumberg 1993). Through the 20th century, the views of menstruation moved from disease prevention to the more formalized social hygiene movement, to commercialization; throughout, the educational materials and consumer appeals segregate menstruation from the topic of sexual activity. The AMA's 1913 publication advances the medicalization of menstruation.

BIOMEDICALIZATION & FEMINIST STS PERSPECTIVES ON HOW MEDICAL TECHNOLOGIES CHANGE SOCIAL RELATIONS, INSTITUTIONS, AND BELIEFS ABOUT WHAT IS NORMAL

Biomedicalization Theory

Adele Clarke (2003; 2010) and her colleagues, seeing limitations of the medicalization framework (Zola 1972; Conrad 1975) in 21st-century medicine, provide a comprehensive theory of biomedicalization. The historical shift from the era of medicalization to the era of biomedicalization crosses several registers, including economic, risk and surveillance, technoscience, knowledge production, and identity creation. Biomedicalization includes five main processes: "major political economic shifts; a new focusing on health and risk and surveillance biomedicines; the technoscientization of biomedicine; transformations of the production, distribution, and consumption of biomedical knowledges; and transformations of bodies and identities" (Clarke et al. 2010, 57). Within these processes, technoscientific applications, or medical technologies, can contribute to identity formation in multiple ways: by helping one to attain a social identity, by imposing performances that enact new subjectivities, by creating new health-related identity categories, and/or by providing new modes of interaction for patients and communities to acquire and perform new identities (Clarke et al. 2010). Clarke's (2010) healthscapes encompass the visual culture of biomedicine, foregrounding high-tech interventions and patient decision-making:

> Healthscapes are ways of grasping, through words, images, and material cultural objects, patterned changes that have occurred in the many and varied sites where health and medicine are performed, who is involved, sciences and technologies in use, media coverage, political and economic elements, and changing ideological and cultural framings of health, illness, healthcare, and medicine. (Clarke et al. 2010)

Biomedicalization theory leans heavily on Foucault's poststructuralist genealogical approach of examining how expertise creates regimes of social control, wherein disciplining governance practices exert biopower over populations (Foucault 1978). Riska (2010) explains that for Foucault power is discursive, meaning there is always resistance, which fits the biomedicalization thesis regarding the emphasis it places on interconnected and multi-directional processes. Additionally, the genealogical approach of tracing when facts and knowledge become fixed and universalized is useful for tracing the emergence of medical knowledge (Riska 2010). Foucault (1978) develops his concept of biopower by examining disciplinary powers such as an anatomo-politics of the human body and regulatory controls, as forming a biopolitics of population; he frames biopower as a development of capitalism and examines institutions of power and techniques of power in the social body.

Rabinow (1996) defines biosociality, an important concept in biomedicalization and biopower. Rabinow uses the emerging human genome project (since he's writing in 1996) to question how our social and ethical practices will change, discussing how new groups and individual identities will be formed through new concepts of risk and genetic testing. Hacking (2005) builds upon Rabinow's biosociality to discuss the formation of new biosocial identities due to genetic risk factors; advocacy and support groups create people and identities. Biomedicalization theory, with its focus on technoscience, healthscapes, biopower, and identity formation, provides a substantive analytical framework from which to analyze new medical technologies, shifting norms, and the production of new subjectivities.

STS Perspectives on Negotiating What's Normal: Medical Technologies

In addition to biomedicalization theory, Feminist STS perspectives provide a breadth of analyses of medical technologies' impact on women's bodies and normalization. Charis Thompson (2001) examines changing beliefs about kinship in fertility clinics. New assistive reproduction medical technologies prompt everyday people to redefine and negotiate new definitions of motherhood by considering genetics, affinity through carrying a fetus, and intention. Here, the flexibility and interconnectedness of the natural and the cultural must be negotiated due to advances in technoscience (Thompson 2001); importantly, it is not that technologies are shaping social norms, but rather it is an interconnected and multidirectional process, which is at the center of biomedicalization. For example, it is now normalized to consider a woman who seeks assistive reproductive technology and carries the fetus the mother, even if genetically she may be unrelated, a sibling, or an aunt. This definition of motherhood considers intent and use of medical technology, illustrating the interconnectedness of the social and "natural" (biological). New technologies incite new negotiations, and norms evolve over time.

Similarly, norms around the use of contraceptive technologies have evolved. Many scholars have examined the interplay between social meanings of contraceptive technologies and bodies themselves, enacted upon by such technologies (Clarke 1998; Mamo and Fosket 2009; Murphy 2012; Takeshita 2012); these analyses will be explored further later in this chapter. In addition, Thompson (2005) and Waldby Cooper (2009) look at how the biological and social are mutually dependent in fertility clinics and stem cell industries, important sites of medical technologies. Thompson (2005) discusses how naturalization and socialization contribute to normalization, defining naturalization as "the rendering of states of affairs and facts in a scientific or biological idiom and to the means by which aspects of the site are rendered unproblematic and self-evident in the sense of seeming 'natural'" (81). For example, once the use of in vitro fertilization is rendered unproblematic and a natural choice, the use of the technology and new definitions of parenthood have been normalized. Waldby and Cooper (2010) look at the stem cell industries, with a focus on labor theory and how women negotiate their roles within the technology and practices of the industry. Regulation and rhetoric shape how women engage with the work, the reproductive practices Waldby and Cooper term regenerative labor. Technologies of stem cell research open up new negotiations around the bioeconomy and feminized labor (Waldby and Cooper 2010). Changing norms around reproductive labor, regenerative medicine, and the potential of the body are negotiated within the context of new biomedical technologies.

Menstrual Scripts and Menstrual Suppression Technologies

In addition to exploring how medical technologies have influenced changing beliefs around kinship, contraception, and reproductive labor, feminist scholars from many disciplines have explored changing beliefs about menstruation. Emily Martin's (1987; 2001) groundbreaking book, *The Woman in the Body: A Cultural Analysis of Reproduction*, examines how medical metaphors and representations exert power and control over women's bodies; conceptions are governed by the limits of language. Martin examines how cultural assumptions and gendered language inform the creation of scientific knowledge, challenging the scientific view of menstruation as failed reproduction; scientific beliefs about normal and abnormal menstruation are illustrated in the definitions and criterion of premenstrual syndrome (PMS). Martin challenges the perception that women are "malfunctioning" (123) and instead challenges the organization of society—specifically, a hyperfocus on productivity and assumed social roles of women. In addition, Martin analyzes in-depth interviews with women about their experiences and beliefs about menstruation, childbearing, and menopause—embracing how women's embodiment can oppose and contradict the stories science tells.

Michelle Murphy (2012), in *Seizing the Means of Reproduction*, examines the technoscientific practices of feminist health activists during the 1970s and 1980s. In the fourth chapter, Murphy traces the history of the Del-Em Menstrual Extraction (ME) device, patented by Lorraine Rothman, as an example of the self-governing of reproduction. Although the device may be used for an early abortion, it was also used by women to manipulate the menstrual cycle. Of this agency, Rothman said, "We no longer wait passively for our monthly visitation. We no longer wait for the first days' cramping to pass. We no longer wait the five to seven days for the whole process to stop. [. . .] We choose to have or to not have, when, where and how" (qtd. in Murphy 2021, 160). Comparisons can be drawn between the empowerment message in the Del-Em informational brochures and the Seasonale advertisements from the early 2000s (Mamo and Fosket 2009). Menstrual Extraction is an example of a layman's medical device to manipulate the menstrual cycle, illustrating the DIY social activism and drive for bodily autonomy evident during this time (e.g., self pelvic exams).

When the pill first hit the market in the United States in 1957, it was not approved as a contraceptive but for gynecological disorders such as excessive menstruation; however, it marked the beginning of a market industry of hormonal manipulation of the menstrual cycle. Nothing prevented off-label use, so the popularity of the pill for contraception boomed. The pill, marketed as Enovid, was then approved for contraceptive use by the FDA in May 1960, and within two years 1.2 million American women were taking it, by 1956 over 6 million (Tone 2021). Because researchers (and the Catholic Church) believed women considered monthly menses "natural" and would be disturbed by the absence of bleeding, the original pill was formulated with 21 days of hormone pills and 7 days of placebo pills, to allow for monthly withdrawal bleeding, to simulate monthly menstruation (Tone 2001; Ghazit 1999; Takeshita 2012). This formulation illustrates the technological construction of "normal."

Direct-to-consumer (DTC) advertising of pharmaceuticals in the United States presents a unique healthscape intersecting popular culture, medicine, and regulation. Many scholars have analyzed the transformation of menstrual scripts in DTC pill advertising, from a focus on preventing pregnancy to a focus on menstrual suppression, including the changing definitions of "period" and bleeding; for example, a "period" while on the pill is now recognized as withdrawal bleeding, not natural menstruation (DeMaria et al. 2019; Kissling 2013; Mamo and Fosket 2009; Hasson 2020). The Seasonale campaign (the first pill marketed for menstrual suppression in 2003) produced cultural scripts about what is normal, transforming monthly bleeding on the pill (withdrawal bleeding) into something unnatural and abnormal, distinguishing between the menstrual period (natural) and the pill period (unnatural and unnecessary) (Mamo and Fosket 2009). If the pill period is not necessary, wouldn't life be more convenient without it? Within a focus on convenience and improved lifestyle emerges the theme of controlling menstruation.

A lifestyle drug is designed to improve the body, rather than treat or prevent disease. Many scholars have examined the shift in advertising and cultural understandings of the pill, from a contraceptive to a lifestyle drug (Watkins 2012; Kissling 2013; Mamo and Fosket 2009). The purpose of the pharmaceutical becomes transformation of the body, optimizing the body for its daily activities. Mamo and Fosket (2009) analyze the production of gendered cultural scripts and feminine embodiment produced through Seasonale advertising materials from 2003–2004. Seasonale is at once a medical discourse and a technocultural intervention, altering women's understanding of what's possible. Kissling (2013) takes this thread further, interrogating the motivations behind this bodily optimization, arguing that these DTC discourses create the neoliberal woman subjectivity, where the subject is expected to make a rational choice for bodily optimization, to create a body that conforms to patriarchy and the neoliberal economy.

DTC advertising for menstrual suppression birth control pills attempted to challenge and shift women's understandings of what a "period" is, differentiating between withdrawal bleeding from hormones and actual menstruation. For consistency of understanding and communication, and for improved research science, regulatory and clinical bodies needed to codify these distinctions as well. Hasson (2020) examines this process, focusing on the development of clinical trial guidelines, developed at the 2005 Hormonal Contraceptives Trial Methodology Consensus Conference, later adopted by the FDA in 2007. Prior to this, clinical trials were inconsistent in measures of and terminology for bleeding. Authors of the new guidelines wanted a focus on timing of bleeding and a distinction between withdrawal bleeding produced by hormonal contraception and actual menstruation (Hasson 2020):

> The use of traditional terminology ("periods" or "menses") should be abandoned with regard to CHCs [combined hormonal contraceptives] and replaced by the use of "scheduled bleeding" or "withdrawal bleeding." E.g., any bleeding or spotting that occurs during hormone-free intervals regardless of the duration of the regimen. "Scheduled bleeding" emphasizes to the woman that her bleeding with hormonal methods is not the same as menstruation. (Mishell et al. 2007, 13, qtd. in Hasson 2020)

Here, bleeding becomes a side effect of the pill. While institutionalizing these new categories of bleeding normalizes menstrual suppression in the clinical world, it is unclear if and how this distinction permeates women's lived experiences.

In a 2007 survey on women's awareness of and beliefs about postponing monthly bleeding, conducted by Szarewski and Moeller (2013), researchers chose to use the term "menstrual bleeding" throughout the survey, for fear that women wouldn't understand the term "withdrawal bleeding." Scholars have evaluated the adoption of menstrual suppression using oral contraceptives in various contexts, including the Hajj pilgrimage (Dandehbor et al. 2016) and the U.S. military (Powell-Dunford et al. 2011). DeMaria et al. (2019), through analyzing interviews and survey data, determine that many women may not understand these distinctions about bleeding or ideas about menstrual suppression. Despite new pharmaceutical, clinical, and regulatory definitions for types of bleeding, it is unclear to what extent these understandings have impacted popular beliefs about monthly bleeding, connection to reproduction, and beliefs about what is healthy or normal.

Although the pill was the first biomedical technology marketed for menstrual suppression, various other products, including hormonal IUDS, include this "side effect" as a potential benefit of using the product. Andrea Tone (1999) argues the IUD is technological violence, critiquing population control strategies that use the IUD as an oppressive form of violent control of passive female subjects, especially among women in low-income countries. Betsy Hartmann makes similar arguments (1995), highlighting how women in the global South did not give consent for insertion, or were denied removal, or otherwise denied proper informed consent; individual women's health and autonomy was put at risk in the service of population-level goals. In *The Global Politics of the IUD*, Takeshita (2012) examines contraceptive research from not only a material perspective but also how scientific work "acts on women's bodies through its discourse" (3). As a politically versatile technology with new discursive arrangements, Takeshita looks at the co-configuration of the IUD and users, grounding the analysis in a Foucauldian perspective of biopower, biopolitical scripts, and the biopolitical subject; broadly, Takeshita argues that the IUD has shifted from a dangerous and oppressive technology to a liberatory consumer product. However, DeMaria et al. (2019) conclude women need to be provided more information about menstrual suppression and IUDs, that understanding "menstrual suppression as healthy and natural" (7) will improve perceptions of hormonal IUDs.

Mirena and Kyleena: Menstrual Scripts and New Norms

Primary Source Selection

Prior research on menstrual suppression has focused on the birth control pill, and prior research on the IUD has often focused on population control and oppression. The intersection of IUDs and menstrual suppression provides a ripe area for analysis. Bayer is the manufacturer and marketer of the Mirena and Kyleena IUDs, and their marketing materials were selected as primary sources for analysis because the Mirena IUD is advertised to "treat heavy periods," and the Kyleena and Mirena IUDs are often advertised together—in web and television advertisements ("Mirena Brochure"). Mirena (available in 2001 in the U.S.) and Kyleena (available in 2016) are levonorgestrel-releasing intrauterine systems, 52 mg and 19.5 mg, respectively. Of the available materials, four television advertisements were selected: a 2013 Mirena ad, 2018 and 2021 ads for Kyleena, and a 2019 ad featuring both Mirena and Kyleena. Both twenty-four pages, the "Mirena Patient Brochure" and "Kyleena Patient Brochure" are PDFs downloaded from Mirena-US.com and

Kyleena-US.com, respectively. Lastly, 2022 web content from WhyIUD.com, Mirena-US.com, and Kyleena-US.com were included.

Methods

Thematic content analysis (or qualitative thematic analysis) was conducted as an iterative open coding process, with a combined inductive-deductive approach. The process involved working from open coding of data to category formation, to development of themes (Seale 2018; Charmaz 2014). To borrow from Seale's (2018) recommendations for discourse analysis, focus was on "1. Identifying key themes and arguments. 2. Looking for association and variation. 3. Examining characterization and agency. 4. Paying attention to emphasis and silences" (486). Secondary sources used to further ground the analysis include Takeshita's (2012) discussion of biopolitical scripts and Clarke's (2010) discussion of biomedicalization and healthscapes.

Descriptive Overview of Primary Sources for Analysis

Bayer provides a patient brochure for both Kyleena and Mirena, available for download from the website, and ostensibly available as a hard copy slick brochure in some medical offices. There are several similarities between both brochures: 1) discussion of *safety* risks, 2) emphasis on *effectiveness* of contraception, 3) emphasis on *size* of the IUD, through text and image, 4) images of smiling women in various contexts, 5) an image of a woman speaking with a female doctor (wearing a white coat and stethoscope). Contrasts between the Kyleena and Mirena brochures include: 1) the way bleeding is discussed and framed, 2) the decision checklist, 3) a redirect page to encourage some readers to research the other product, and 4) the types of images of women, specifically, a) the presence of men (or not), and b) the implied age range of women in the images.

The WhyIUD website links to both Mirena-US.com and Kyleena-US.com. Both websites repeat the information in the brochures and include additional information. The websites are also more interactive than the brochures, as the reader is encouraged to click on tabs or buttons to find targeted information about their interests and concerns. Notably, the Kyleena website includes two personal testimonials from social media influencers in the form of Instagram posts; clicking on the post takes the consumer to the Instagram platform. Both the patient brochures and the websites include substantively more information about periods and bleeding than the television commercials.

The four television commercials provide more developed narrative scenes and more detailed images than the website or brochure sources. The Mirena 2013 commercial focuses on one woman, a mother of a rambunctious toddler, who initially wonders if she forgot to take her pill; the narrative focus in on her busy life and the fact that she does want another child, just not right now; mention of periods only comes at the very end. The Kyleena 2018 commercial provides a more overt focus on heterosexual sexual encounters, showing several women worrying about whether they took or packed their pills, illustrating how one woman solves this problem by getting the Kyleena IUD, appearing empowered and carefree as she meets a man for a date. Both narratives imply that women are forgetful about taking the pill, and both narratives are about taking control but with the help of technology.

The Mirena and Kyleena 2019 commercial serves to compare the two products by showing the stories of two different women: one who cannot keep a houseplant alive (who chooses Kyleena), and another who is already busy with one toddler (who chooses Mirena). In contrast to the other commercials, the Mirena and Kyleena 2019 commercial includes an appeal to community and group membership: "Join the millions of women who have used IUDs like Mirena and Kyleena." Lastly, the Kyleena 2021 commercial is comprised of a rotating montage of scenes of four women: one working in a professional kitchen, one studying in a high school, one preparing in her garage to take a trip, and one leaving and then arriving home to her husband and children. The four narratives all have an overtly sexual and heteronormative focus, each ending with the woman flirting with a man; the overall emphasis is on a woman's contraceptive needs at different stages in life. The patient brochures, television advertisements, and website content all show a variety of races of women and medical professionals, casting a broad representation; class is somewhat ambiguous although what many viewers may interpret as "middle class."

ANALYSIS: KEY THEMES AND SCRIPTS

Characterization of Bleeding: Normalizing Heavy Menstrual Bleeding Needs Treatment

Technological interventions that target broad notions of health can shape new beliefs and understandings, in an iterative process between society and the technologies. Regarding the framing of bleeding and periods, the Kyleena and Mirena IUD materials contrast with the menstrual suppression pill materials. Recall that Seasonale advertising makes a distinction between a real period and withdrawal bleeding (Mamo and Fosket 2009); there is no such distinction made in the IUD materials, which makes sense because the hormone delivery is constant, and many women don't experience any bleeding at all. "Period" is the default term for monthly bleeding, and "spotting" is used to name other bleeding that may occur. In contrast to the Seasonale advertisements, the medical condition "heavy menstrual bleeding" (HMB) is defined and discussed in the IUD materials—a definition that is malleable and flexible. In the IUD materials, Bayer defines for women what is abnormal, or pathological, about a period: heavy bleeding. In contrast to menstrual suppression pill ads where the focus is on normalizing *no period* as a healthy option, whether altering periods is healthy or normal is not stated directly in the IUD materials. However, this claim is implicit in two areas: discussion of *treatment for HMB* and discussion of IUD *side effects*.

Both the IUD patient brochures and websites provide a substantive amount of information on bleeding, in contrast to the television commercials. Both brochures and websites have a similarly formatted header, "How Mirena [or Kyleena] may affect your period" (12, 10). The first section of this page is identical for Mirena and Kyleena, explaining that in the first 3 to 6 months the period may become irregular, and spotting is common. The products are differentiated in the last section. The Kyleena materials state, "For some women, periods will stop altogether," (10) while the Mirena materials state, "By the end of year one, about 20% of users have no period at all" (12). We can deduce that the absence of labeling Kyleena as a therapeutic for heavy periods is due to FDA approvals, not actual device function or material reality.

The Mirena materials foreground treating heavy periods. In large font, the front of the Mirena brochure reads, "Looking for birth control that helps with heavy periods?" (1), and the next page reads, "Effective birth control that helps with heavy periods" (2). The Mirena IUD materials define HMB as an abnormal condition that demands treatment and provide tools (such as lists) to help women self-assess their own menstrual cycle as normal or not. The following definition of HMB is included on the Bayer Kyleena and Mirena IUD brochures and websites:

> HMB is excessive menstrual blood loss (≥ 80 mL, or about 6 tablespoons) during a single cycle. You may have HMB if you:
>
> - Need to double up on pads to control your menstrual flow
> - Have menstrual periods lasting more than 7 days
> - Need to change pads or tampons during the night
>
> Many symptoms can indicate HMB, so talk to your healthcare provider. (Bayer 2022)

The similar list on the website also includes the following two items: "have a menstrual flow that soaks through one or more pads or tampons every hour for several hours in a row" and "have a menstrual flow with blood clots the size of a quarter or larger." If the woman determines she has HMB by using the information on the website, she now has a diagnosis and treatment to name when she speaks with her doctor. The definition of HMB appears subjective, malleable, and perhaps not all that uncommon. Measuring actual blood volume is challenging and not routine, and many women may have had to change a pad or tampon at night. One compelling absence here is the lack of any other corporeal aspect of heavy menstrual bleeding, such as cramps, bloating, migraines, mood disturbances, or other types of discomfort. It's possible that women's primary complaints from HMB may be related to pain and discomfort, rather than the simple metric of blood volume; the last sentence of the HMB definition section of the brochure, "Many symptoms can indicate HMB, so talk to your healthcare provider," opens the door for diagnosis by other clinical observations, or reported symptoms, in the actual healthcare setting.

Interestingly, changes in bleeding due to the use of an IUD are characterized as both a therapeutic treatment and a side effect. Side effect typically denotes an undesirable unintended effect of a medication, but here the side effect of missed menstrual periods is implicitly desirable. Both the Mirena and Kyleena brochures and websites have a similar section that begins, "Common side effects include missed menstrual periods." The subsequent sentence in the Kyleena materials reads, "About 12 out of 100 women stop having periods after 1 year of Kyleena use." The subsequent sentence in the Mirena materials reads, "About 2 out of 10 women stop having periods after 1 year of Mirena use." In contrast to the Kyleena materials, the Mirena materials include a section titled "With Mirena, your heavy periods may change," accompanied by a graphic illustrating an 80 percent reduction in bleeding after 3 months and a 90 percent reduction in bleeding after 6 months. The Mirena brochure notes that "Mirena rapidly reduces heavy periods," (9) followed by clinical trial data. In contrast to the websites and brochures, the television commercials do not focus on bleeding. The Mirena 2013 ad includes the following statements, "Periods over time may become shorter, lighter, or may even stop" and "Did you know, if you choose Mirena to prevent pregnancy, it's also approved to treat heavy periods?" highlighting heavy periods as a condition worthy of treatment. The other three commercials share this identical language: "Bleeding and spotting may increase in the first three to six months and remain irregular. Periods over time may become lighter, shorter, or may stop," stated in a neutral way and not framed as either a benefit or side effect.

Both brochures and websites include a flowchart titled "Which IUD birth control is right for me?" with two lines that follow: 1) "I want an IUD that will also help with my heavy periods," or 2) "I want a 5-year IUD with a low dose of hormones." Although there is not explicit discussion of normalizing having no periods, there is a rhetorical move to normalize *the use of the device* through references to the numbers of women who use it, a group appeal. The Kyleena brochure says, "Millions of women have already used IUDs—including women who have had a baby and those who haven't" (3). The Mirena brochure says, "Mirena is the #1 prescribed IUD in the U.S." (3). The 2019 combined Mirena and Kyleena commercial encourages, "Join the millions of women who have used IUDs like Mirena and Kyleena."

The Medical Device: Technological Object in the Healthscape

The IUD as medical device is a material-semiotic object (Haraway 2004); it possesses concrete material characteristics and functions as a medical technology; it also produces meaning, transforming not only the body but understandings and beliefs. Healthscapes may be understood as cultural landscapes with material and symbolic registers, as assemblages or infrastructures, as images, as items, as assumptions. Clarke connects healthscapes to Foucauldian recursive regimes, where media and images do the work of legitimation (Clarke 2010). The primary sources chosen here act within the current healthscape by providing distinct cultural framings of women's lives and concerns, defining contraception options, defining heavy menstrual bleeding as deserving of treatment, and framing woman's biosocial identity (Hacking 2005) as one of options, choice, and agency. Ultimately, women are consumers of biomedical goods and practices; making choices amongst these goods requires negotiating myriad risks (as articulated in all pharmaceutical ads in the U.S.), possibilities, effects, and requires self-surveillance. Examples of self-surveillance include monitoring a pill regimen and the body's response to a new pill, or manually checking IUD strings.

In this instance, the technological object in the healthscape is a medical device, the IUD, present on websites and television commercials, and even social media platform campaigns. Three themes emerge from the primary sources about the IUD as technological object: 1) focus on material aspects of the device (size, materials, distinct medical imagery of device and women's anatomy, how it works), 2) medical procedure for acquiring the device, and 3) efficacy of the device compared to other contraceptive methods.

The brochures and websites both show a similar image of the IUD "actual size" next to a common household object and size specification. The Mirena IUD is shown next to two stacked dice and is 1.26 inches. The Kyleena IUD is shown next to earbuds and is 1.18 inches. Materials for both highlight "small and T-shaped" and "soft, flexible plastic." This same image is shown on a tablet a female doctor holds in the combined Kyleena and Mirena 2021 commercial. Similarly, the 2013, 2018, and 2019 television ads contain an image of a hand holding the device between the thumb and forefinger, pressing lightly to illustrate the flexibility, and the narration includes words such as "small" and "effective." The flexibility and small size imply the object's unobtrusiveness to the body. The annotated images of the device within the uterus, in the brochures and websites, serve to further demystify the placement of the device. The brochures and websites include a section titled "What to expect during placement." The materials also foreground the contraceptive efficacy of the device, the websites and brochures all including the same vertically oriented graphic with the top arrow labeled "More effective: Greater than 99%" and the lower arrow labeled "Less effective: Approx. 70%." The top row includes the arm implant, IUD, injections, and sterilization. The next row down includes the pill, patch, and ring; the next down includes condoms and diaphragm; the bottom row includes spermicides and withdrawal. The television ads emphasize efficacy with phrases such as "reliable," "low maintenance," "over 99% effective," and "highly effective." "Low maintenance" implies the IUD requires less self-surveillance than the other methods. The depth of information provided, along with images, solidifies the device in the healthscape and serves to normalize the IUD as a smart consumer choice.

Subjectivities

Women's Roles: Contrasts and Absences

Women are depicted in various roles in the IUD materials, including mother, wife, student, worker, and woman dating. The characterization of women's roles is most developed in the TV ads, as the medium allows illustration of scenes and implied context quickly with visual elements. The 2013 Mirena commercial focuses on one woman, a mother to an active toddler, navigating various scenes of daily life. Through narration, the woman expresses that she doesn't want to have to remember a pill every day, and that she does want another child but not now. The 2018 Kyleena ad shows three different young women, ostensibly childless, navigating heterosexual intimate encounters; the focus in on how Kyleena will take the worry, about forgetting to pack or missing pills, away. The 2021 Kyleena ad is similar but the four women in this montage illustrate heterosexual women's need for contraception at four different stages of life. The narratives of all four women follow a similar thread by ending with a man in the last scene, showing that this IUD can be used across a lifetime of menses, an expansion of biomedicalization. The first woman is a young professional chef working in a kitchen (man is coworker); the second woman is a student diligently studying in what appears to be a public high school (man is another student); the third woman is a Jeep and dog owner packing her car in her garage for a trip (man appears to live there also and is going on the trip); the fourth woman is a nurse who has a busy home with two kids and a husband. The 2019 ad comparing Mirena and Kyleena focuses on two women and their different needs, one woman who can't keep a houseplant alive, implying she shouldn't become pregnant, and another woman who already has one child and would like to wait before having another.

Similarly, we can see contrasts in women's roles in the patient brochures. Although the Mirena brochure has one image of a man and woman within, the cover image is three women of varying ages, outdoors, smiling; the image on the back of the brochure is a woman smiling with her child. There is no implication of sex on the front or back of the Mirena brochure. In contrast, the Kyleena brochure shows images of heterosexual implied intimate relations on the front, back, and interior of the brochure. The three women shown on the front of the Kyleena brochure also appear younger as a group, compared to the Mirena brochure. Although the brochures do provide substantive information about the therapeutic use of the Mirena IUD for heavy menstrual bleeding (HMB), the subjectivities of women illustrated either state or imply that women's primary desire for the device is contraception, a need illustrated by the heterosexual intimacy scenarios; this heteronormative focus produces a gendered subjectivity for the imagined ideal consumer for the product. Absent from the representations in these materials are non-heterosexual women and trans men who might also desire treatment for HMB. Would lesbians and trans men not also appreciate access to a low-hormone treatment for heavy menstrual bleeding?

Scripts: Choice and Practice of Self

In addition to women's roles, we can further examine the production of subjectivities through these DTC advertising materials, considering productivity, responsibilization, optimization, agency, choice, and practice of self. Takeshita (2012) identifies three biopolitical scripts of the IUD over time: *population*, *choice*, and *the practice of self*. These scripts capture how technologies, users, and modes of bodily governance are configured together. Second-wave feminist movements and beyond illustrate the fight for women's individual contraceptive choice and bodily autonomy, illustrating the biopolitical script of choice. Individual biopolitical subjects are encouraged to take personal responsibility for contraceptive choice, as evidenced in the Kyleena patient brochure: "Plan on your own terms," and "Choosing birth control is personal" (3). Consumers are encouraged to make this choice for themselves on the IUD websites: "You know what makes sense for yourself. So when it comes to birth control, you should go with what makes sense for your life and your body." Throughout the IUD materials, women are encouraged to choose between the pill and IUD as the only smart choices for contraception. The Kyleena website states, "1,826 daily pills over 5 years vs. 1 Kyleena IUD" and "eliminates the responsibility of taking a daily pill." Further, women are encouraged to choose between Kyleena and Mirena, based on whether they want a treatment for heavy menstrual bleeding, even though both devices have similar effects on reducing bleeding. Takeshita argues that since menstrual suppression pills already solidified menstrual suppression as a lifestyle choice, viewers are willing to accept a "major side effect" (139) as bodily enhancement. Enhancing one's body, through use of the device, can be understood as optimization; enhancement contrasts with a fix for a specific medical condition (HMB). Women can choose their contraception type, and they can also choose to enhance or optimize their bodies.

The discourse of choice shapes the practice of self. Takeshita argues that the rhetoric of rights can be viewed as self-governance in free societies, under the broader expansion of responsibilization, of managing and controlling one's body, within a liberal capitalist society: "The biopolitical script of a free society consists of the 'practice of self,' or self-governance, facilitated by the discourses of choice" (29). Takeshita's practice of self dovetails with Clarke's (2010) "tailoring of the self via transformations of embodiment, enmindedment, and enselfment (especially via drugs)" (24). Treating heavy menstrual bleeding and eliminating a daily pill will enhance one's lifestyle, while treating HMB will also enhance one's bodily functions. Throughout the IUD materials, we can see that an optimized body, whether optimized to avoid pregnancy or reduce HMB, brings smiles, confidence, and contentment to the subjects shown. Evaluating whether one has HMB that needs treatment requires a reflexive self-surveillance with the aim to optimize one's life and body. In this script, understanding and acting on the choice to get an IUD requires a sense of agency to make positive change. The possibility for change is realized in the advertising: the Mirena brochure asks, "Did you know? Mirena is the #1 prescribed IUD in the U.S." and the Kyleena brochure asks, "Ready for a birth control that doesn't require a daily routine?" These questions indicate the reader may be missing out on something to further optimize their health and life; the questions pique the readers' interest; engaging with those answers engages with the practice of self. However, unlike the pill, a doctor must medically insert the IUD and take it out; in some ways, this is less control.

The practice of self script is developed within the Instagram testimonials posted on the Bayer Kyleena website. Scrolling down the main page of the website brings the viewer to "Hear what some influencers have to say about Kyleena, and how it makes sense for them, and fits into their life!" The encouragement to evaluate what will enhance one's life prompts the practice of self. Yolande Kelly's Instagram testimonial, by @yolandekelly:

> Thinking about adding a dog to the family one we're in the new house . . . but that's it for now. I rely on my Kyleena [. . .], a reliable, low-maintenance birth control option with no daily pills to remember. So, every day for up to 5 years, I don't have to remember to take a daily pill. (Kelly 2022)

Tatum Dahl's Instagram testimonial, @tatedoll:

> A big part of what makes me so driven to be open online is the fact that my following predominantly consists of women who want to make informed decisions. Because of this I feel strongly about sharing my own personal experiences, especially the important ones. Learning about the @Kyleenarx IUD was one of the best decisions I have ever made for myself! I believe that information is power and allows you to choose what is best for you. (Dahl 2021)

Dahl's Instagram testimonial praises her audience for wanting to make informed decisions and encourages them to do what is best for them. Implicit in her statement that learning about the Kyleena IUD "was one of the best decisions" she has ever made is that it might be the best decision for her followers as well. "Information is power" encourages her followers to feel empowered and follow through with looking further into the device. In contrast, Kelly's Instagram testimonial focuses on the convenience of not having to take a daily pill, optimizing her body for her daily routine. Kelly's post most clearly illustrates the choice script, outlining the choice between the IUD and pill. Dahl's post more explicitly engaged with the practice of self. In both cases, readers may feel a sense of agency to investigate this product that might help them optimize their bodies.

In sum, the discourses in the Mirena and Kyleen IUD materials present a malleable and flexible definition of HMB, giving consumers a tool for identifying and naming the medical condition. Additionally, the materials frame menstrual suppression as both a treatment for HMB and a simple side effect of the IUD contraceptive choice; implicit is the possible lifestyle benefit from such bodily optimization or enhancement, of having one's period stop altogether. Here the IUD, as a material-semiotic object in the healthscape, contributes to a technological construction of normal by framing menstrual suppression as a normal choice many women make, a smart choice. The discourses within these materials encourage women to identify as an HMB sufferer and/or identify with the millions of other women who have chosen an IUD, shaping new biosocial identities. The biopolitical script practice of self demonstrates and constructs new definitions around menstrual bleeding; these discourses produce a gendered subjectivity of responsibilization and agency, encouraging optimization of the body within a discourse of choice.

Topics for Further Research

While this analysis adds to the existing literature around IUDs as medical technology and the emergence of menstrual suppression as a consumer choice, several areas call for further research:

- What are the changing demographics of IUD users in the U.S., by age, race, and socio-economic status (SES)?
- What are the popular and social beliefs about IUDs, amongst women of varying demographics (age, race, SES) in the U.S., regarding availability, efficacy, access, safety, and risk?
- How is the definition of heavy menstrual bleeding (HMB) used clinically? For example, the definition is based on volume of blood, which is hard to determine; for many women, the more relevant medical concern may be pain and discomfort.
- How do women's beliefs and understandings of menstrual suppression differ for various populations or demographics? To what extent does the average woman understand the difference between menstruation and withdrawal bleeding, or menstrual suppression as a consumer choice option?
- Currently, the U.S. and New Zealand are the only countries that allow DTC marketing of pharmaceuticals and devices. Is there a difference between how menstruation is medicalized, or not, between these countries and other Western countries without DTC advertising?

MENSTRUAL FUTURES

In 2015, runner Kiran Gandhi made headlines when she chose to freebleed during the London Marathon. The iconic photograph, with the crotch area of her legging stained dark red, was circulated online, garnering both praise and disgust. The story was covered by *Cosmopolitan, The Independent, Vice, The Daily Mail* (Jung 2015; Barnes and London 2015; Gandhi 2015; Bona 2016). That same year, controversy erupted online when Instagram removed (twice) a photo of a fully clothed woman on her bed, which showed blood stains on her pants and bedsheet; Rupi Kaur, a Canadian artist working to break taboos around menstruation, posted the image (Holden 2015). Like menstrual suppression, or skipping periods, has been normalized by medical and pharmaceutical discourses, visible bleeding, or at least discussion of it, may be becoming less taboo. Additionally, menstrual activists publicly interrogate the access and affordability of menstrual care products, arguing for health and education equity for people around the world (Carney 2020;

Crawford et al. 2019; Haneman 2021; Bakibinga et al. 2021). Due to this visibility and activism, several states and countries have eliminated taxes on menstrual care products. Broadly, a public consciousness has coalesced that promotes visibility, demystification, choice, access to care, and agency over one's body. Each menstruator (whether woman, trans man, or nonbinary individual) can choose for themselves and attempt to augment their body's bleeding with the help of various medical technologies; this choice, and optimization, has become normalized as a practice of self. Under the neoliberal framework of responsibilization, denaturalizing female bodily processes has become naturalized.

Medical technologies for menstrual suppression are here to stay, but DeMaria questions whether patient-consumers have a full understanding of these technologies (2019). Further research must be conducted to assess menstruators' lived experiences and beliefs, in addition to their understandings of scientific and medical definitions, mechanisms, and recommendations. In addition, in many states in the U.S., the overturning of *Roe v. Wade* has opened a field of new political and legislative interventions and infringements on menstruators' lives. Contraception and menstrual management are two reasons menstruators choose to adopt these medical technologies, but increasing government surveillance may newly inform and shape those concerns. These concerns are not held by only cishet women as portrayed in the Kyleena and Mirena advertisements; contraception and menstrual management are concerns of all people who menstruate.

Further research must be conducted to ascertain the effects of new legislation on the adoption of long-acting reversible contraceptives (LARCs), such as IUDs, over the pill. Through the discursive practices of this historical moment, what new subjectivities will be produced? What will this mean for practices of the self? Within these research areas, scholars should remain attuned to examining stratified access to affordable medical care, medical technologies and choices, and consumer knowledge about those choices.

REFERENCES

Bakibinga, Elizabeth and Nightingale Rubuka-Ngaiza. 2021. "The Role of Addressing Poverty and Inequality in High Income Countries: A Comparative View of Menstrual Hygiene Management and Its Impact on Education and Health in the UK and Select High Income Sub-Saharan African Countries." *Law & Development* 14.2: 503–549.

Barnes, Sarah and Bianca London. 2015. "'Women's Bodies Don't Exist for Public Consumption': Runner Hits Back at Critics after Being Branded Disgusting for Completing London Marathon During her Period without a Tampon." *Daily*

Mail. https://www.dailymail.co.uk/femail/article-3201878/Runner-completed-London-Marathon-free-bleeding-hits-critics-uncomfortable-normal-process.html

Bayer. 2022. "Kyleena." Kyleena-us.com. Accessed November 2022. Kyleena-us.com

Bayer. 2021. Kyleena 2021 March TV Spot, downloaded November 2022: https://ispot.tv/a/OwNt, also here: https://www.kyleena-us.com/

Bayer. 2018. Kyleena 2018 May TV Spot, downloaded November 2022: https://ispot.tv/a/dkcP

Bayer. 2022. "Kyleena Patient Brochure." PDF downloaded November 2022. Kyleena-us.com

Bayer. 2022. "Mirena." Mirena-us.com. Accessed November 2022. Mirena-us.com

Bayer. 2019. Mirena and Kyleena 2019 February TV Spot, downloaded November 2022: https://ispot.tv/a/Ilr7

Bayer. 2022. "Mirena Patient Brochure." PDF downloaded November 2022. Mirena-us.com

Bayer. 2022. "Why IUD." WhyIUD.com. Accessed November 2022. https://www.whyiud.com/

Bona, Emilia. 2016. "Freebleeding in Sports: Fighting the Tide Against the Menstruation Taboo." *Vice.* Vice Sports UK. https://www.vice.com/en/article/bmqvvd/freebleeding-in-sports-fighting-the-tide-against-the-menstruation-taboo

Brumberg, Joan Jacobs. 1993. "Something Happens to Girls: Menarche and the Emergence of the Modern American Hygienic Imperative." In *Women & Health*, 150–171. (Originally published in *Journal of the History of Sexuality* 1993).

Bullough, Vern and Martha Voght. 1973. "Women, Menstruation, and Nineteenth-Century Medicine." *Bulletin of the History of Medicine*, 47.1: 66–82.

Carney, Mitchell O'Shea. 2020. "Cycles of Punishment: The Constitutionality of Restricting Access to Menstrual Health Products in Prisons." *Boston College of Law Review*, 61.7: 2541–2594.

Charmaz, K. 2014. *Constructing Grounded Theory* (2nd Edition). London: Sage.

Clarke, Adele. 1998. *Disciplining Reproduction: Modernity, the Life Sciences, and the Problems of Sex.* University of California Press.

Clarke, Adele et al. 2003. "Biomedicalization: Technoscientific Transformations of Health, Illness, and U.S. Biomedicine." *American Sociological Review*. 68.2: 161–194.

Clarke, Adele et al. 2010. *Biomedicalization: Technoscience, Health and Illness in the U.S.* Durham: Duke University Press.

Clouston, T.S. 1883; 1884. "Female Education from a Medical Point of View." *Popular Science Monthly*, 24: 322–333.

Conrad, Peter. 1975. "The Discovery of Hyperkinesis: Notes on the Medicalization of Deviant Behavior." *Social Problems*. 23.1: 12–21.

Crawford, Bridget J. et al. 2019. "The Ground on Which We All Stand: A Conversation about Menstrual Equity Law and Activism." *Michigan Journal of Gender & Law*. 26.2: 341–348.

Creswell, J. W. 1994. *Qualitative Inquiry and Research Design*, Thousand Oaks, CA: Sage Publishing.

Dahl, Tatum. @Tatcdoll. "#BaycrPartncr #WhyKylccna." Instragram.com/p/CVyOzdTvWWJ/ Posted 2 November 2021. Accessed November 21, 2022.

Dandehbor, Wealeed et al. 2016. "Menstrual Suppression Using Oral Contraceptives by Female Hajj Pilgrims." *The International Journal of Travel Medicine and Global Health*, 4.4: 111–114.

DeMaria, A.L. et al. 2019. "The Myth of Menstruation: How Menstrual Regulation and Suppression Impact Contraceptive Choice." *BMC Women's Health*, 19:125.

Dewey, John. 1886. "Health and Sex in Higher Education." *Popular Science Monthly*, 28: 606.

Foucault, Michel. 1978. *The History of Sexuality*, Vol. 1. Pantheon Books.

Gandhi, Kiran. 2015. "Here's Why I Ran the London Marathon on the First Day of My Period – and Chose Not to Wear a Tampon." *Independent.* https://www.independent.co.uk/voices/comment/here-s-why-i-ran-the-london-marathon-on-the-first-day-of-my-period-and-chose-not-to-wear-a-tampon-10455176.html

Ghazit, Chana. 1999. "The Pill." PBS, *American Experience*.

Hacking, Ian. 2005. "Genetics, Biosocial Groups & the Future of Identity." *Daedalus* Fall: 81–95.

Haneman, Victoria J. "Menstrual Capitalism, Period Poverty, and the Role of the B Corporation." *Columbia Journal of Gender & Law*, 41.4: 133–145.

Haraway, Donna J. 2004. "Morphing in the Order: Flexible Strategies, Feminist Science Studies, and Primate Revisions." *The Haraway Reader*. Routledge: 199–222.

Hartman, Betsy. 1995. *Reproductive Rights and Wrongs: The Global Politics of Population Control.* Boston: South End Press.

Hasson, Katie Anne. 2020. "Not a 'Real' Period?: Social and Material Constructions of Menstruation," in C. Bobel et al., eds., *The Palgrave Handbook of Critical Menstruation Studies*. Palgrave Macmillan.

Holden, Steven. 2015. "Instagram Period Photo: Woman Who Took It Says She Wasn't Being 'Provocative.'" *BBC News.* https://www.bbc.com/news/newsbeat-32105388

Jung, Helin. 2015. "26-Year-Old Woman Free Bleeds Proudly Through Her First Marathon." *Cosmopolitan.* https://www.cosmopolitan.com/health-fitness/q-and-a/a44392/free-bleeding-marathoner-kiran-gandhi/

Kellogg, J. H. 1882. *Plain Facts for Old and Young*. I. F. Segner.

Kelly, Yolande. @yolandekelly. "#BayerPartner @Kyleenaapi." Instagram.com/p/CcnKG-xrELu/ Posted 21 April 2022. Accessed November 12, 2022.

Kissling, Elizabeth Arveda. 2013. "Pills, Periods, and Postfeminism: The New Politics of Marketing Birth Control." *Feminist Media Studies*, 13.3: 490–504.

Mamo, Laura, and Jennifer Ruth Fosket. 2009. "Scripting the Body: Pharmaceuticals and the (Re)Making of Menstruation." *Signs* 34: 925–949.

Martin, Emily. 1987; 2001. *The Woman in the Body: A Cultural Analysis of Reproduction*. Beacon Press.

Maudsley, Henry. 1884. *Sex in Mind and in Education*. C. W. Bardeen.

McMillan, Colleen, and Amanda Jenkins. 2016. "'A Magic Little Pill that Will Relieve You of Your Womanly Issues': What Young Women Say About Menstrual

Suppression." *International Journal of Qualitative Studies on Health and Well-Being*, 11: 32932.

Murphy, Michelle. 2012. *Seizing the Means of Reproduction: Entanglements of Feminism, Health, and Technoscience.* Duke University Press.

Powell-Dunford, Nicole C. et al. 2011. "Menstrual Suppression for Combat Operations:

Advantages or Oral Contraceptive Pills." *Women's Health Issues*, 21.1: 86–91.

Rabinow, Paul. 1996. "Artificiality and Enlightenment. From Sociology to Biosociality." *Essays on the Anthropology of Reason*. Princeton, NJ: Princeton University Press.

Renault, Marion. 2020. "No One Has to Get Their Period Anymore: Menstruating is Painful, Expensive, and . . . Unnecessary?" *The Atlantic*. July 2020. https://www.theatlantic.com/science/archive/2020/07/why-menstruate-if-you-dont-have/614350/

Riska, Elianne. 2010. "Gender and Medicalization and Biomedicalization Theories." *Biomedicalization: Technoscience, Health and Illness in the U.S.* Durham: Duke University Press. 147–172.

Seale, Clive. 2018. *Researching Society and Culture* (4th Edition). London: Sage.

Szarewski, Anne and Cecilia Moeller. 2013. "Women's Perceptions about Reducing the Frequency of Monthly Bleeding: Results from a Multinational Survey." *Open Access Journal of Contraception*, 2013.4: 29–37.

Takeshita, Chikako. 2011. *The Global Biopolitics of the IUD*. MIT Press.

Thompson, Charis. 2001. "Strategic Naturalizing: Kinship in an Infertility Clinic," in Sarah Franklin and Susan McKinnon, eds., *Relative Values: Refiguring Kinship Studies*, 175–202. Durham: Duke University Press.

Thompson, Charis. 2005. *Making Parents: The Ontological Choreography of Reproductive Technologies*. MIT Press.

Tone, Andrea. 1999. "Violence by Design: Contraceptive Technology and the Invasion of the Female Body," in Michael A. Bellesiles, ed., *Lethal Imagination: Violence and Brutality in American History*. New York: New York University Press.

Tone, Andrea. 2002. *Devices and Desires: A History of Contraceptives in America*. Farrar, Straus and Giroux.

Waldby, Catherine, and Melinda Cooper. 2010. "From Reproductive Work to Regenerative Labour: The Female Body in the Stem Cell Industries." *Feminist Theory* 11.1 (2010): 3–22.

Walt Disney Studios. 1945. *The Story of Menstruation*.

Walt Disney Studios. 2022. *Turning Red*.

Watkins, Elizabeth Siegel. 2012. "How the Pill Became a Lifestyle Drug: The Pharmaceutical Industry and Birth Control in the United States Since 1960." *American Journal of Public Health*, 102.8: 1462–1472.

Zola, Irving Kenneth. 1972. "Medicine as an Institution of Social Control." *Sociological Review*, 20: 487–504.

Chapter 6

The Emporia of Aristotle

What Prosthetics Taught Us About the Human Body

Alan Hawk

The earliest known prosthetic limbs date from Roman times. One artificial limb discovered in an archeological excavation near Capua, Italy, dated from approximately 300 BCE. Deterioration of the artifact that left just a bronze sheath and fragments of wood prevented any effort to reconstruct the device, evaluate its effectiveness as an artificial limb, or determine how it functioned. The artifact was destroyed due to a bombing raid during World War II.[1]

The artificial limbs from the Renaissance were peg legs that were more functional on a patient who survived a below-knee amputation than one above the knee. One artificial limb described by Ambroise Parè (1510–1590) could be unlocked to be bent at the knee when the wearer either sat or mounted a horse. When the wearer wanted to walk, he locked the joint into a configuration of a peg leg.[2] William Harvey's (1578–1657) observation in 1615 that blood ran through a closed circulatory system gradually transformed conventional wisdom about blood loss, leading to Jean-Louis Petit (1674–1750) developing the tourniquet about a century later to control hemorrhage. This instrument increased the chances of a patient surviving amputation, thus increasing the demand for prosthetic legs.[3]

A prosthesis is the merger of the human body with the mechanical, the animate with the inanimate. Probably the first published English definition of the term *prosthesis* was in 1706: "In surgery prosthesis is taken for that which fills up what is wanting. . . . Also the making of artificial legs and arms when the natural ones are lost."[4] The loss could be acute, either caused by a bullet, a shell fragment, or a machine, or by a gradual loss of function through arthritis or degenerative bone disease. Its design is informed by what prosthetists, surgeons, and/or biomedical engineers understood about how what they were replacing really functioned and of what they thought they were attempting to replace. It requires the replacement of skin, bone, muscle, ligaments, and tendons, with its elastic and flexible properties, by a material with very different characteristics, such as wood, metal, leather, rubber, ceramics, and composite materials. Some prostheses attempt to mechanically replace the function of the part, while some attempt to recreate the form of the part; and, finally, others are a combination of both.

More than most medical interventions, a prosthesis defines an individual's identity and self-image. It is the first step of healing and is where the patient relearns how to walk. It is the line between self-sufficiency and dependency. It is something to be hidden or displayed prominently. It is something to be explained every time the person goes through airport security. Its serial number is useful in identifying the body after death. By the twenty-first century, there are prosthetics to replace any part of the body that could be wanting; everything from heart valves to elbow joints to blood vessels to the inner ear. Given the scope of this topic, this chapter will focus on how prostheses taught us how the lower extremities function.

In the early nineteenth century, Scottish surgeon John Bell (1763–1820) was one of the first professors to teach medical students the relevance of anatomy to the practice of surgery. He described the skeletal structure in one volume of his textbook *Engravings of the Bones, Muscles and Joints*, and the muscles that articulate the limb in the other. His explanation of the skeletal system divided the lower limb into the thigh (defined by the femur), the leg (defined by the tibia and fibula), and the foot. The relationship of these sections was not defined, and the knee was described as either surfaces of the tibia or the femur rather than as a joint. Only in his description of the muscles does he describe the lower limb as a single entity. Since surgeons of this era could do little more than debride wounds and amputate limbs, perhaps it is not surprising that he doesn't discuss the lower limb as a functional unit.[5]

After the loss of his own leg, James Potts,[6] a clockmaker of Belford, England, invented one of the first of these lower limb prostheses at the turn of the nineteenth century: "The knee and ankle are entirely at the command of the wearer; and the appearance of their motions is so natural, as very nearly to conceal the loss of the extremity. . . . The wearer can kneel and rise up; can sit down and rise up; can pull on a boot, . . . ride on horseback with perfect safety, and imitate almost any motion without any assistance of his hands." Potts claimed he could walk eight to ten miles a day without fatigue.[7] The prosthetic gained notoriety when Henry Bayly (1768–1854) was wounded during the battle of Waterloo in 1814, resulting in the amputation of his right leg, and subsequently was fitted with one of these artificial limbs. He became

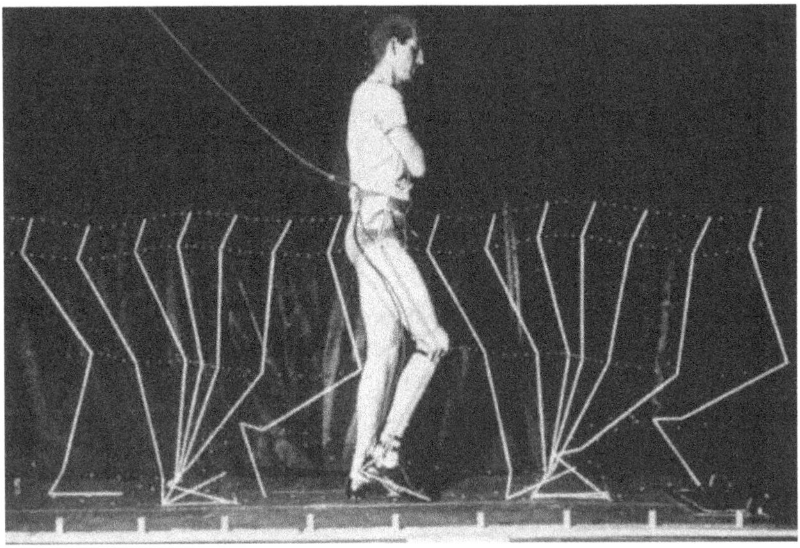

Figure 6.1. Subject walking showing lines drawn through corresponding positions at the University of California, Berkley, published in 1947 by University of California at Berkley (National Research Council).

the first Marquess of Anglesey a year later and, as a result, Potts' artificial limb became known as the "Anglesey leg."[8] The device articulated at the knee and had a stop to prevent it from hyperextending. The momentum of the passing phase provided the forward swing of the leg. The ankle joint was a brass ball and socket. A foot carved to look like a human foot had a piano hinge to allow a separate block carved in the shape of toes to flex while walking. The spring of the toes was provided by the shoes worn over the foot.[9] The Anglesey leg spurred demand for more functional artificial legs, as opposed to the peg leg, and led to the continued development of more lifelike prostheses with bendable knees and flexible feet that permitted the wearer to walk with a reasonably normal gait.

The gait cycle is an analysis of human locomotion. There are two distinct, but simultaneous, phases in walking: the swing, or passing phase, and the support phase, or mid-stance.

1. The swing phase is when one leg moves forward in preparation for the next step. Heel-off is when the foot rotates onto the toes, followed by toe-off, which pushes the leg to lift off the ground, move past the other leg, and contact the ground, called heel strike.
2. The support phase leg bears the weight of the body while the other leg is in the swing phase. After heel strike, the foot lands flat as the leg

transitions vertically to support the body and then rocks forward to heel-off and continue the cycle.

Anatomical movement of the leg is described in the following terms: extension increases the angle of the joint, such as straightening a bent leg. Flexion decreases the angle of the joint, such as bending a straight leg. Rotation is the movement of the limb along its vertical axis resulting in turning the foot inward (medial rotation) or outward (lateral rotation).

If a leg bows outward from the midline of the body, it is described as valgus, and if it angles inward, it is described as varus.

The product of a tradesman stimulated questions in academia. Throughout the eighteenth and early nineteenth centuries, several physiologists occasionally commented on the process of walking, but performed no experiments to test their theories. The experts in mechanics believed walking was primarily driven by gravity, while those trained in physiology assumed muscular activity.[10] An example of the latter was published by physician Archibald Robertson (1789–1864) in 1827:

> Supposing the person is in erect posture, to walk forward at an ordinary pace, it is performed by first bending one thigh upon the pelvis, straightening the leg raising the foot from the ground, and thus producing a general shortening of the limb, which advances it forward; then the limb rests upon the ground, first touching with the heel, and successively the whole anterior parts of the foot. During this time, the pelvis rotates upon the thigh upon the head of the limb which is immoveable; carrying forward the whole limb which is raised from the ground, and that whole side of the body. As yet there is no advance; the limb which is behind is brought forward in the following manner: the foot behind is detached from the heel to the toes, by a movement of rotation, of which the centre is the articulation of the metatarsus with the phalanges, so that towards the end of this movement, the foot does not touch, except by these last; the limb is lengthened, the trunk is carried forward, by rotating the pelvis on the head of the thigh formerly carried forward.[11]

Robertson served as a Royal Navy surgeon during the Napoleonic Wars (1803–1815). His emphasis on the role of the pelvis pulling apparently passive legs to move forward was suggestive of a person wearing an artificial limb, rather than the complex interplay of bone, muscle, and ligament.

In 1836, Wilhelm Weber (1804–1891) and Eduard Weber (1795–1881) conducted a series of experiments to measure the mechanics of locomotion, which they published in their treatise *Mechanik der menschlichen Gehwerkzeuge*. They timed several individuals walking a known distance and calculated phases of their stride. Using human skeletal lower limb specimens, they attempted to deduce the range of motion to create a mathematical model on how humans walked. Their calculations of stride length, frequency, and the up-and-down movement while walking as well as inclination of the body in motion were ultimately recognized as accurate. However, the more theoretical aspects of their research, those that were harder to measure, such as the actual movement of the limb, resulted in a distorted depiction of human locomotion. Because of their assumption that the leg behaved like a pendulum, similar to the motion of the Anglesey leg, they had the subject's leg swing freely to simulate the passing phase. Calculating the range of motion using bones without muscle and ligaments exaggerated the degree of flexion and extension.[12]

Unlike Bell's depiction of the human leg as its shape and the sum of its parts, both Robertson's and the brothers Weber's accounts were an effort to describe how the lower limb functioned. It was an attempt to understand the act of walking: a common phenomenon that people had taken for granted. While neither discussion references the artificial limb, it is perhaps significant they occurred after its invention.[13]

One of Potts' protégés, William Selpho (1811–1890), emigrated and became the first manufacturer of artificial limbs, based on the Anglesey leg, in the United States. One of his patients was Benjamin Palmer of Meredith, New Hampshire, who, at the age of 10, had his leg crushed, resulting in amputation. The artificial leg proved problematic for Palmer, and he discarded the leg and then used a crutch, which also proved challenging. Having struggled with two possible solutions to his condition, he set about developing a third. Palmer received the first U.S. patent for an artificial limb on November 4, 1846, described as "improved articulations of the knee, ankle and toes." The knee flexed on a highly polished bolt. A "tendon" cord ran from the top of the calf through the hollowed limb to just forward of the ankle pin on which the foot, a wood block shaped to the contours of a human foot, pivoted. The purpose of the tendon was to make sure that the lower limb did not hyperextend during the forward swing of the leg during the passing phase. Another block of wood carved to serve as the toes pivoted on a third hinge pin.[14] Perhaps the best tribute to Palmer's design was the award of one of the 2,913 prize medals from the 1851 Great Exhibition in London, the only artificial limb so honored at the event by the nation that had invented the leg prosthesis.[15]

When journalist Oliver Holmes (1809–1894) visited Palmer's prosthetic workshop in 1863, the story he wrote became a discourse on how people walk. He described one of the workers carving out the socket, who turned out to be an amputee who wore an artificial leg. He was asked to walk across the room to determine which leg was "nature's leg" and which was Mr. Palmer's. Still not certain, he was asked to walk back and forth again. After considerable deliberation, Holmes guessed the wrong leg.[16]

Holmes described the process of walking, possibly one of the first published attempts at gait analysis. The movements of the legs were compared to the movement of a pendulum, a construct that did not allow for rotation of the limb. Comparing research on locomotion gained in the laboratory by anatomists versus observation of how people walked in the community, Holmes observed:

> The mathematical formulae in which the Messrs. Weber embody their results would hardly be instructive to most of our readers. The figures of their Atlas would serve our purpose better, had we not means of coming nearer to the truth than even their careful studies enabled them to do. We have selected a number of instantaneous stereoscopic views of the streets and public places of Paris and of New York,[17] each of them showing numerous walking figures, among which some may be found in every stage of the complex act we are studying.[18]

Although not a complete picture, he could piece together the basic stages of locomotion. He outlines the basic stages of the gait cycle (see figure 6.1), perhaps for the first time accompanied by illustrations taken from the images. He concluded:

> Walking, then, is a perpetual falling with a perpetual self-recovery. It is a most complex, violent, and perilous operation, which we divest of its extreme danger only by continual practice from a very early period of life. We find how complex it is when we attempt to analyze it, and we see that we never understood it thoroughly until the time of the instantaneous photograph.[19]

However, in the 1840s, Palmer could only rely on his observations of people going about their daily business to design his artificial limb.

Trauma as a consequence of industrialization spurred the development of artificial limbs. Improved surgical technique ensured that the patient was more likely to survive the procedure. The number of people requiring amputations after their legs were accidentally crushed increased with the introduction of machinery in farms and factories along with railroad vehicles and streetcars. Soldiers sustained severe wounds from improved firearms and munitions in major wars such as the Crimean War (1853–1856), Second Italian War of Independence (1859), the American Civil War (1861–1865) and the Franco-Prussian War (1870–1871). As a result of the Civil War, American soldiers received 3,798 lower limb prostheses from ten separate manufacturers between 1862 and 1866. State governments of the former Confederacy and private charities such as the Association for the Relief of Maimed Soldiers provided artificial limbs to wounded veterans. In 1866, the state of North Carolina estimated the need for 550 prosthetics for their soldiers.[20]

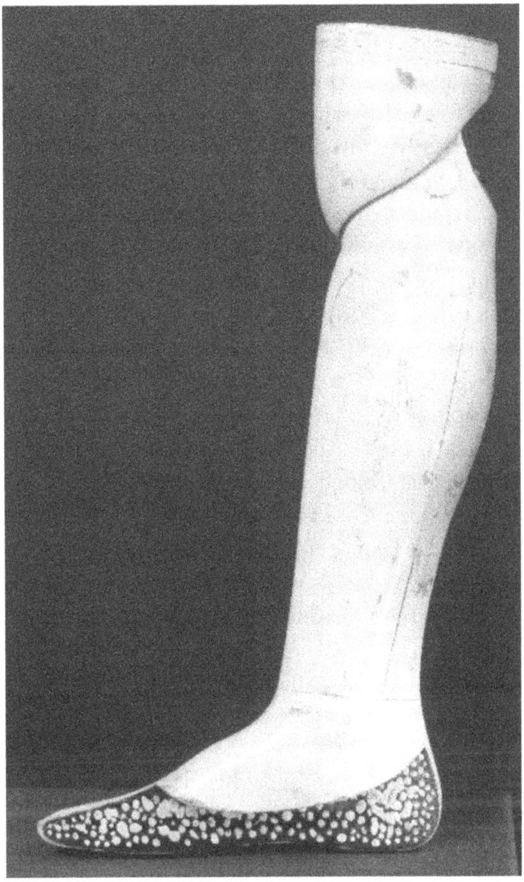

Figure 6.2. Model of A. A. Marks artificial limb featuring the rubber foot. Plate on model reads "Model artificial leg for thigh amputation Marks Patent rubber foot imitated in wood and shown in section" [M-129.00060] (Disclosure: This image has been cropped to emphasize the subject.) (National Museum of Health and Medicine photo by Matthew Breitbart/Released)

Another prosthetist, Amasa Marks (1825–1905), began manufacturing artificial limbs in 1853. The ankle joint of his prosthetic limb used an adjustable spring to orient the foot during the passing phase prior to heel strike. However, after devoting much of his practice to repairing these ankle joints, Marks concluded that another approach was required. In 1863, he was awarded a patent on a foot constructed of India rubber. The foot was composed of sponge rubber and a harder substance, either hard rubber or wood, that would be attached to the prosthesis (see figure 6.2). The patent claimed, "The natural movement of the foot is more closely imitated by my improvement than by any other before known, while at the same time the cumbrous, expensive, and delicate attachments ordinarily used to effect [sic] the same purposes are dispensed with."[21] Later versions were reinforced with metal spring steel bars in canvas embedded in the rubber foot.[22]

Meanwhile, there were several efforts to measure the process of locomotion. One of the first systemic analyses of how people walk was defined by French scientist Étienne-Jules Marey (1830–1904) and published in the 1870s.[23] His measurements of a person walking relied on a single sensor on the foot that indicated pressure on the foot while in motion. It was used to determine how long feet were on the ground. Another system measured the up-and-down motion of the body while underway.

Eadweard Muybridge (1830–1904) was hired by Leland Stanford (1824–1893), president of the Union Pacific Railroad, to settle a bet. Stanford needed to prove that a galloping horse, at times, lifts all four feet off the ground and hired Muybridge to take photographs to prove his assertion. With Stanford's patronage, Muybridge developed a camera battery that took a sequence of photographs while the subject was in motion and proved that Stanford's horse Occident indeed lifted all four feet while in full gallop.[24]

In 1883, Muybridge was hired as part of the faculty of the University of Pennsylvania in Philadelphia to continue his work generating a series of now iconic images of people, clothed and nude, performing a variety of tasks. Three years later, he generated 786 plates consisting of 122,436 individual images breaking down motion into separate steps. While two of these surviving plates feature amputees (plate 537 features a man who had sustained a single amputation of a leg, hopping with crutches, and plate 538 shows a boy who had sustained a double amputation at his thighs), none showed the subject wearing a prosthesis.[25]

As the nineteenth century progressed, Marks' clientele transitioned from wounded soldiers to victims of industrial accidents. The individuals likely to need an expensive prosthesis were men and women of modest means. He was selling the ability to walk again, and he needed to demonstrate that the expense was worthwhile, since an amputee could resume his profession. As a result, his company published a series of books that were a compilation how people had used their limbs to overcome misfortune. Each book included a chapter on gait analysis with illustrations clearly inspired by Muybridge's plates. Developing the rubber foot raised questions that inspired further study of the process of locomotion, first through photographs (1888) and later through motion film (1914). Marks noted the knee had greater flexion as a person's pace increased, while that of the ankle decreased. A wooden artificial foot hampered a person's ability to walk greater than three miles per hour, since the sole of the foot was on the ground longer than the natural foot. The compressibility of a rubber foot allowed the sole to remain on the ground for a period comparable to a natural foot. Marks' artificial limb set the pattern for artificial limbs into the late twentieth century.[26]

There were many accounts in popular culture during the late nineteenth century of how effective the prosthetic limbs were in restoring patient mobility. Holmes described his inability to discern which of the workers at the Palmer factory were wearing artificial limbs. Marks included testimonials in his books. James McDonald, who lost both legs below the knee due to a railroad accident, testified to his ability to ride a bicycle, ice skate, and dance at parties. William Harms described working as a baggage master at a train station in Parksville, New York, and carried a trunk that weighed more than 125 pounds on his shoulder. Four-year-old Ambrose Mullen, a double amputee at the age of two, running on his artificial limbs, was almost indistinguishable from the other children with whom he played. Carrie Kuntz, who sustained an amputation at the age of seven, grew up, got married, and was "the fond mother of an interesting family." Professor F.E. Jacoby was able to resume his profession as a tightrope walker after being fitted with a Marks artificial limb.[27] The American monthly *Galaxy* dryly observed in 1871:

> Your morning mail is swelled . . . by circulars of various artificial limb-makers, giving diagrams of sundry legs, and testimonials of people who have walked, danced, and run better than ever with them. You almost gather the impression that it would be better to be born with legs, arms, and head perhaps, all wood, ready patented—a second Frankenstein.[28]

While the prosthetic limb technology was assuming the form it would take for the next half century, German surgeon Themistocles Gluck (1853–1942), after a decade of experimentation on animals, implanted the first artificial knee joint in a 17-year-old girl on May 20, 1890. The prosthesis was made of ivory, which was selected for its supposed similarity to bone, thus likely to better integrate the femur and tibia. Thirty-five days after the procedure, he reported to the Berlin Medical Society that the patient was pain free and had a relatively good range of movement of the leg. Despite Gluck's stringent aseptic technique, postoperative infection caused the prosthesis to fail. The lack of success ensured that knee arthroplasty would not be attempted until the 1940s.[29]

On January 19, 1945, Sgt. Dewey Force (1921–1989) became one of 5,482 soldiers who had sustained a lower limb amputation due to combat during World War II. He wrote to his parents the next day, recovering from surgery: "I am feeling pretty frisky tonight. Another operation in a week or so and I should be ready for one of those factory-made feet."[30] The below-knee artificial limb he received was similar to the limb manufactured by Marks, a plywood leg with a rubber foot. He was fitted with the limb a week before he was due to be married, which motivated him to learn to use the leg so that he could walk to the altar and greet his bride standing on his two feet, unaided by crutches. After the war, he became a professor of special education and an advocate for people with disabling conditions, arguing, "The emphasis should be on what a person has, not what he has not."[31]

To improve the rehabilitation of soldiers like Force, the University of California, Berkeley, received a grant from the Committee on Prosthetic Devices of the National Research Council for an interdisciplinary team of engineers, physicians, and anthropologists to characterize human locomotion in order to provide background information to improve artificial limbs issued to amputees. They evaluated the importance of the rotation of the leg in the rhythm of walking in normal individuals, discovering that the average rotation of the pelvis during the walking cycle was 8.0 degrees, the femur was 15.2 degrees, and the tibia 19.3 degrees, with an average value of 9.1 degrees as the relative rotation of the tibia with the femur. Medial rotation occurred when the knee was fully extended as the leg transitioned vertically and lateral rotation as it transitioned to toe-off. The description of the process of walking had evolved from the impressionistic account of Robertson into one that was quantifiable. The difficulty in quantifying the process of walking before photography was that Robertson described medial rotation as occurring prior to toe-off, while Berkeley observed that it occurred between mid-stance and toe-off.[32]

Experience in treating many cases allowed for a more nuanced understanding of standing and locomotion, based on the comparison of amputees wearing his or her prosthesis with individuals retaining both their original limbs. Even when standing, a person remains upright through active stability, as his or her torso sways slightly in relation to the ankle joints, with the hip typically forward of the ankle. With an artificial foot, the rigid ankle shifted the axis of rotation toward the toes. For the person to stand normally, the instep of the artificial foot had to carefully set, otherwise the leg would either lean forward or backward when weight bearing, causing the upper body to counterbalance, thus disturbing the alignment of the body and making it difficult for the patient to maintain balance.[33]

The loss of a limb is extremely distressing to an individual, disrupting his or her confidence. One disorienting effects is the persistent, sometimes painful, feeling that the removed limb still exists. Although the phantom limb was first observed by American surgeon and pioneering neurologist S. Weir Mitchell (1829–1914) while treating wounded soldiers at Turner's Lane Hospital in New York City during the Civil War, the significance to a person's ability to use an artificial limb became apparent in the post–World War II era. "Its value to the amputee is enormous," British neurologist Michael Kremer (1907–1988), dean of the Associated Institute of Neurology in London,

England, observed, "I am quite certain that an amputee with an artificial limb can walk on it satisfactorily until the body image, in other words, the phantom is incorporated into it." Oliver Sacks, professor of Neurology and Psychiatry at Columbia University in New York City, described how one of his patients woke up his phantom limb by flexing his thigh stump and slapping it before putting on his artificial limb and walking.[34] After an individual's sense of self has been disrupted by the loss of the limb, he or she needs to integrate the loss of limb, phantom pain, and introduction of the prosthesis into their new body image. This process was inadvertently described by Bennett Wilson, technical director of the U.S. Committee on Prosthetics Research and Development: "The phantom sensation usually recedes to the point where it occurs only infrequently or disappears entirely, especially if a prosthesis is used."[35] Younger individuals have greater difficulty integrating the prosthesis, generally a result of trauma, since they are more likely to see it in terms of lost life opportunities. In contrast, older amputees who are more likely to have sustained the loss due to a chronic condition tend to see it in terms of increased mobility. For it to work, the wearer needs to mentally incorporate the prosthesis into his or her body.[36]

Meanwhile, Austin Talley Moore (1899–1963) was implanting the first successful joint prostheses when he replaced the proximal end of the femur with a metal appliance that matched the form of the hip. A 52-year-old African American man had a tumor at the neck of the right hip that caused severe degeneration of the bone. In 1940, after years of conservative treatments had failed, Moore inserted a Vitallium hip implant. Upon recovery, the patient had regained 75 percent of normal hip function and was able to walk with a cane. When he died two years later from an acute heart attack, the prosthesis was extracted and found to be in excellent condition.[37]

Moore resumed designing his artificial hip in 1950. The original design was modified to move the femoral neck into a more anatomically accurate position (see figure 6.3). In the first half-decade of his procedure, he reported success with his first 153 patients, a majority of whom were 60 to 70 years old. One 74-year-old housewife who had an acute hip fracture, identified as Mrs. T.P., was able to walk with a moderate limp assisted by a cane. Mrs. I.M., a 51-year-old mill worker diagnosed with arthritis, was able to walk unassisted with a slight limp and, presumably, resume her career. Mr. L.H., 72, who sustained a hip fracture that would not heal, was able walk with a slight limp, assisted by a crutch.[38]

It should be noted that since joint prostheses are developed and implanted by surgeons, their description of outcomes differed from those of prosthetists. Artificial limbs were marketed to the amputee through narrative descriptions of individuals who had recovered from similar experiences, using the advertised product. Artificial joints were marketed to other physicians, relying on

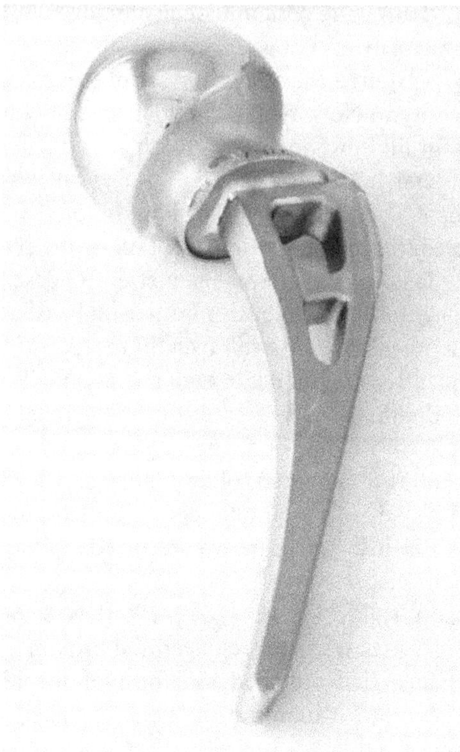

Figure 6.3. This is an Austin Moore Hemi-Hip prosthesis manufactured by Howmedica, Inc., in the 1970s. This type of prothesis was invented by J. Austin Talley Moore (1899–1963), orthopedic surgeon at the Moore Orthopedic Clinic at Colombia University in New York City and first implanted in 1950. [M-129.11109] (Disclosure: This image has been cropped to emphasize the subject.) (National Museum of Health and Medicine photo by Ian Herbst/Released)

clinical and statistical descriptions of outcomes that they could use to compare to similar products to make informed recommendations to their patients.

The implantation of the large metal appliance didn't cause a toxic reaction inside the human body nor was it subject to loosening.[39] On the contrary, compression resulting from weight bearing of the prosthesis caused thickening of the bone around the implant. German anatomist and surgeon Julius Wolff (1836–1902) posited in 1892 that bone will remodel itself according to the load placed upon it.[40] Perhaps this was the first practical application of this theory, which had become known as "Wolff's Law." Austin Moore's rehabilitation protocol with the patient standing, assisted by a crutch, on the limb with the hip prosthesis provided the necessary compression by weight bearing to facilitate healing. He recommended that patients use a cane, minimize weight gain, and "advised to avoid excessive stress in the same way that one who uses a dental prosthesis avoids excessive chewing of hard or tough food."[41] Of the 55 patients Moore had followed up with after two years, 45 had good to excellent outcomes defined as being able to walk unaided, or assisted with a crutch or a cane, and having a slight or moderate limp with a complete range of motion.

The Austin Moore hip replaced only the femoral head and not the acetabular socket, and the prosthesis could not produce the synovial fluid needed to lubricate the joint. British orthopedic surgeon John Charnley (1911–1982) realized that the prosthesis needed to replace both the femoral head and the acetabular socket. Unlike his predecessors, he looked at the artificial hip as an engineering problem as well as a medical problem. He designed the stainless-steel hip with a smaller ball joint than found on a human hip that fitted into a high-density polyethylene plastic acetabular socket. The smaller ball joint allowed for a thicker socket and friction comparable to the synovial lubrication of the normal human socket. He was the first to use cement to fix the prosthesis to the bone. The first Charnley Low-Friction artificial hip was implanted in January 1960. A five-year follow-up by Charnley of his first 138 cases demonstrated that 96 percent of the patients obtained pain relief and 84 percent had improved mobility.[42] Although other designs for the artificial hip have been developed, it is remarkable that both designs remain in production more than a half-century after invention.

The hip proved to be a relatively simple prosthesis to develop, as it was a copy of the joint it was intended to replace, albeit in a modified form by Charnley. The success of the hip prosthesis gave surgeons confidence that the knee would be equally easy to copy. Gluck had set the pattern for knee prosthesis development assuming, as did the creators of artificial limbs, that the knee functioned like a hinge.

After World War II, a variety of orthopedic surgeons followed Gluck's concept of the knee as a hinge. One of the first was Swedish surgeon Börje Walldius (1913–1998) of the Karolinska Institutet, Sweden, who implanted his first artificial knees in 1951. The first examples were a hinge joint made of steel-reinforced acrylic; later versions were made of stainless steel. While these efforts initially appeared to be successful with a good range of motion of the leg, the knee joint proved to be more complicated than the simple hinge that these surgeons had envisioned.[43]

To improve upon these prostheses, a multinational consortium known as the Groupe pour l'utilisation et l'étude des prothèses articulaires (GUEPAR) formed at the Pavillon Ollier, Hôpital Cochin in Paris, France, and quickly settled on developing a hinge knee. To more closely duplicate the motion of the joint, the group moved the pivot of the hinge joint closer to the knee's natural axis of rotation, allowing for greater flexion. One of the prostheses from the first production batch was tested under two criteria for resistance to wear

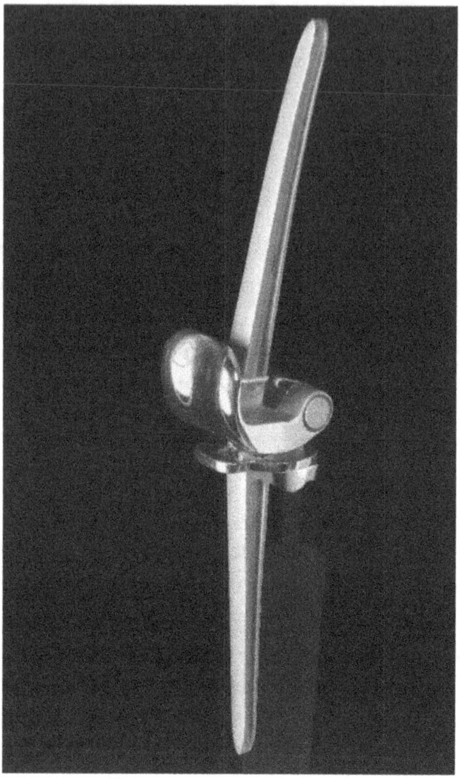

Figure 6.4. The GUEPAR Total Knee, also known as the Offset Hinge Total Knee, was introduced in 1970. The prosthesis had a high failure rate since it was a solid metal linkage that lacked the impact absorbing structure of the meniscus of the normal human knee joint. The rigid hinge joint did not allow the flexibility of medial rotation of the joint whilst walking. This knee was removed by Hospital for Special Surgery in New York, New York. [M-129.10071] (Disclosure: This image has been manipulated using dodging and burning techniques. It has been cropped to emphasize the subject.) (National Museum of Health and Medicine photo illustration by Matthrew Breitbart/ Released)

and biomechanical behavior by cycling the prototype to 120 degrees flexion at 70 cycles per minute under a load of zero to 100 kg (more than 220 lbs.). Since only 0.237 mm of wear was noted at the hinge after 1,000 hours of testing without any apparent degradation to the prosthesis, wear seemed quite acceptable.[44]

The first GUEPAR Offset Hinge prosthesis was implanted in October 1969 (see figure 6.4). In the subsequent five years, the GUEPAR Consortium implanted artificial knees in 292 patients, mostly women, a majority (65%) of whom were between the ages 65 and 85. The general health of the cohort can be deduced by complications during surgery: five sustained cardiac arrest;

eight had respiratory insufficiency; and 12 suffered from neurovascular problems. Approximately 17 percent of the patients sustained problems resulting from the difficulty in performing an experimental surgical procedure, ranging from damage to the bone and tendons, to deep wound infections and loosening of the prosthesis within the first year. However, outcomes were promising as all patients reported improvement in walking ability resulting from increased stability and relief from pain; 93 with decreased pain, while 63 were pain free. The prosthetic allowed for a flexion of 90 degrees in 85 percent of the cases and 120 degrees in 26 percent.[45]

However, the optimistic prognosis was based on short-term results. In 1976, John Insall (1930–2000) of the Hospital for Special Surgery in New York City concluded that the GUEPAR knee had the best outcomes two to three-and-a-half years postoperatively compared with the non-constrained knees coming onto the market, although the apparently glowing endorsement included an important caveat: "It must be emphasized that in this study, we did not attempt to determine the long-term survival rate of any of these prostheses. Our follow up was too short for that purpose and it may well be that by the end of five years our results will be very different than they are now."[46]

The problem with hinge knee prostheses, of which the GUEPAR knee was the most sophisticated iteration, was their inflexibility. Theodore Waugh (1926–), Chief of the Division of Orthopedic Surgery, University of California, Irvine, proposed another solution, one that duplicated the form of the articular surfaces and preserved the interior cruciate ligaments. After multiple designs were evaluated and discarded, the result was the UCI Total Knee replacement with a Vitallium femoral component replacing the condyles of the knee and a thin tibial tray made of polyethylene. A series of cutting guides ensured accurate placement of the prosthesis. Like the GUEPAR knee, outcomes were promising at first. Of the first 25 cases, preoperative patients moved using crutches or wheelchairs with the average range of motion of 64 degrees. In the 28 weeks after the procedure, all patients reported a complete lack of pain and were able to move with less support than prior to the operation. One patient was able to walk unaided an average of four miles a day. Patients suffering from bilateral knee problems inquired when the other knee could be replaced.[47]

Short-term results did not mean positive long-term outcomes. Surgeons noted problems two to three years after implantation, where the failure rate was commonly 30 to 35 percent. One study found that 73.5 percent of these prostheses failed five years after surgery. But by 1979, surgeons were communicating with each other that "routine use of the GUEPAR valgus-hinge knee was unacceptable."[48] The UCI knee fared little better. In 1982, Dr. Lynne Hamilton of the Ochsner Medical Institutions in New Orleans, Louisiana, concluded in a follow-up study that one-fifth of the UCI knees implanted by the surgeon had required further surgery. Apparently, the posterior cruciate ligaments pulled the prosthetic condyles toward the rear, thus lifting and separating the front end from the bone. Since the tibial component was only 5 mm thick and was pliable, it became loose and subsided into the bone softened by the disease. Eight of those prostheses were later revised with a GUEPAR knee.[49] Neither approach, whether replacing the knee joint with a hinge or carefully cutting away the damaged joint surfaces in order to replace the joint surfaces, turned out to be successful.

How the human knee functioned was imperfectly understood when both prostheses were being developed and questions about the stress sustained by the human knee had not been asked, let alone answered. In 1967, James Morrison completed his doctoral dissertation, "The Forces Transmitted by the Human Knee Joint During Activities," where he described his measurements of the stresses borne by the knee during routine activities:

> Forces acting across the articulating surfaces of joints have recently received much attention due to their importance in the design of internal prostheses and in the understanding of joint lubrication problems. The external force system acting at the knee joint has been measured by several researchers: Elftman (1940), Marks and Hirschberg (1958), Bresler and Frankel (1950). Total force acting across the joint, however, has not been investigated in detail prior to the present study.[50]

He determined that the articulating surface of the tibia sustained a force of 3.4 times the body weight just during level walking. The anterior cruciate ligament sustained a force of approximately 35 pounds and the posterior cruciate ligament bore 74 pounds. Ascending a flight of stairs imposed a force of 4.25 times the body weight, which is not a constant force, but a pounding felt every time the foot touched the ground. The maximum load occurred immediately after heel strike and shortly after heel-off.

In the late 1970s, Edmund Chao (1938–) of the Mayo Clinic in Rochester, Minnesota, used sensors to analyze the preoperative and postoperative gait of individuals receiving artificial knees, a twentieth-century version of the research pioneered by Marey. The subject wore shoes with five binary sensors to measure which part of the foot was in contact with a stainless-steel floor mat to measure stride length and width. A force plate measured reaction force between the foot and the floor, while optical switches measured velocity. A triaxial electrogoniometer simultaneously measured knee joint flexion and rotation. Subjects were also tested on steps and a 15-degree ramp. This system measured a definite functional improvement of the joint one year after total knee replacement.[51]

The GUEPAR Consortium, as did all involved with hinge prosthesis designs of the period, failed to appreciate that a solid metal linkage lacked the impact absorbing structure of the normal human knee joint. It failed to consider the rotation of the leg while walking. The biomedical engineers at the University of California, Irvine, did not consider the stresses on the prosthetic tibial tray. The early confidence illustrated by Walldius in 1951 concluded in an article on his knee prosthesis:

> It is interesting from the mechanical and biological point of view to compare the conditions for endoprosthesis operations in the hip and knee joints. . . . In the knee joint, the weight bearing is at a right angle to parallel even surfaces without the same degree of lever effect as in the hip joint. . . . It is therefore evident that the conditions for successful results of operations with endoprosthesis are greater in the case of a knee joint than in a hip joint.[52]

The early confidence was shattered by the realization of how little was understood about this joint and the determination to study the biomechanics of the knee. More than 20 years later, a humbler Chao reflected, "No other joint in the human body is as demanding as the knee joint, since it must be adaptable to large stresses and still maintain a high degree of mobility, as well as stability. These functional requirements predispose the design conditions for prosthetic devices."[53]

An application of the lessons learned was a new generation of artificial knees developed by Insall in 1974. The Total Condylar Prosthesis featured a 25 mm thick polyethylene tibial tray to absorb the impact of walking. The design required the removal of the cruciate ligaments to simplify the procedure but did not compensate for their removal. Although a successful implant was made, surgeons sometimes made errors during installation, causing laxity in the joint. Only a quarter of the patients could ascend stairs correctly. In 1978, Insall partnered with biomedical engineer Albert Burstein (1937–) to develop the Posterior Stabilized Condylar Prostheses to correct this deficiency. A spine was incorporated in the tibial tray to stabilize the joint, replacing the function of the cruciate ligaments. The cam on the femoral component is in contact with the spine which stabilizes the artificial joint. Of the first 118 knees implanted in the first year, 88 percent were rated as excellent two to four years later with stable and painless joints. The worst-case scenario was that elderly patients needed the assistance of a banister to climb stairs.[54]

Insall conducted another survey to determine the long-term effects of total knee replacement. He reported that, after an average of 6.6 years post procedure, 91 percent of the outcomes were either good or excellent. "The best testimony of all," Insall concluded, "was that most patients stated that they had forgotten that they had a knee prosthesis."[55] Perhaps this is also an example of a person mentally incorporating the prosthesis, albeit an implant, into his or her body.

As prosthetic joints were being perfected, new materials and technology transformed the development of artificial limbs. Improved surgical techniques, such as internal fixation of fractures, vascular surgery, and nerve repair, increased the chances of a patient retaining his or her limb. In the nineteenth century and first half of the twentieth century, prosthetics treated patients that sustained trauma, either by war or industrial accident. By the twenty-first century, trauma accounted for only 20 percent of amputations and most amputations were performed to treat vascular diseases, such as diabetes.

Composite materials allowed for the creation of better-fitting stump sockets and a lighter limb. Hydraulic knee joints replaced the elastic cords of the nineteenth-century and early twentieth-century prosthetics. In 1997, Otto Bock Healthcare introduced the C-Leg microprocessor-controlled knee. The knee is controlled by software algorithms that adapt to the wearer's movement. People fitted with the limb appreciated the capability to adapt to any walking speed. At the beginning of the swing phase, the residual limb had slower flexion speed resulting in a calmer swing of the artificial limb that was better synchronized with the natural movement of the remaining leg. The microprocessor adjusted the movement of the knee while the wearer was in motion, allowing them to adjust their gait according to the circumstances without thinking about it. If a person inadvertently dragged the foot on the ground, one advantage was that the C-Leg resisted buckling, making recovery likely.[56]

Another approach was the blade prosthesis using a carbon fiber spring for the foot, a concept similar to Marks' use of rubber for his feet. Energy was stored from the weight of the wearer during the support phase is released in toe-off. However, the blade prosthesis does not attempt to duplicate the form of the foot, nor does the wearer even try to hide the fact that he or she is wearing an artificial limb. This is the ultimate incorporation of the prosthesis with the body, providing the amputee with a new self-image (see figure 6.5). Despite being a double amputee since he was an infant, Oscar Pistorius (1986–) of South Africa qualified to compete as a sprinter in the 2012 Olympics in London while Markus Rehm (1988–) was denied his chance in 2016 on the grounds that his prostheses gave him an unfair advantage against his "able-bodied" opponents. Perhaps the 1871 observation was correct: it would have been better to have been born with legs of wood, the amputee as a cyborg rather than a cripple.[57]

The use of prostheses to replace losses has become routine. Newer designs of artificial joints use better anatomical configurations, and 3D printing and ceramics continue to move the state of the art forward. Over 90 percent of the artificial knees implanted still function after 15 years. In 2017,

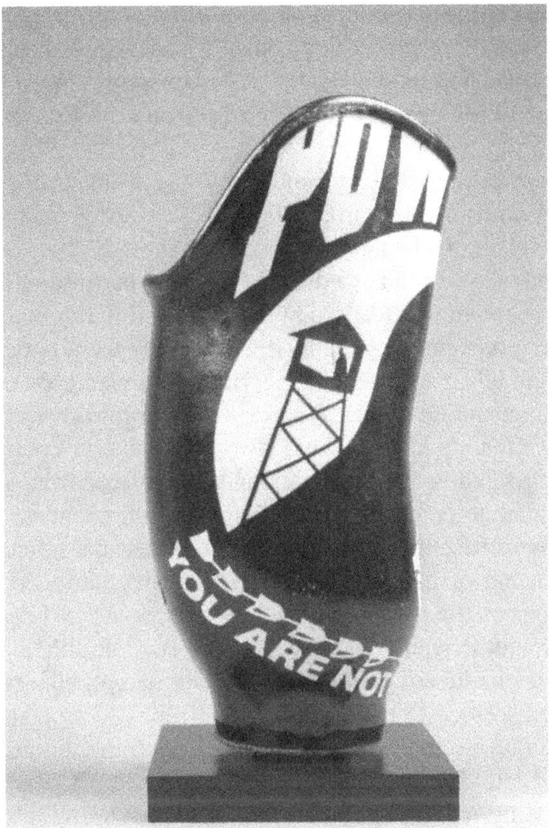

Figure 6.5. Prosthesis Stump Socket, custom made circa 2005, at the Walter Reed Army Medical Center from a 3-D scan of the amputee's residual limb. (M-129.11305) (Disclosure: This image has been cropped to emphasize the subject.) (National Museum of Health and Medicine photo by Matthew Breitbart/Released)

approximately 600,000 knee prostheses were implanted in the United States as were 330,000 artificial hip implants to treat degenerative joint diseases. About seven million people in the United States are living with artificial knee or hip joints.

In contrast to the rapid evolution of artificial joints, artificial limbs have followed more of a punctuated equilibrium model incorporating advances in materials. Robotic feet have allowed amputees to rise on their toes. Another promising technology is osseointegration where the artificial limb is directly connected by a detachable abutment implanted in the femur or tibia. By eliminating the need for a stump socket, amputees are able double the distance they could walk and reduce exertion for the six-minute walk test used to evaluate functional pulmonary and cardiovascular capability of an individual.

Patients reported that an osseointegration prosthesis provided "a much more intimate and 'part of me' experience than a socket prosthesis."[58] In 2017, surgeons performed approximately 185,000 amputations in the United States. Just under two million people who have sustained limb loss are living in the United States.

Consider the meaning of this technology to these nine million people with either artificial limbs or joint prostheses; people who would have been confined to a wheelchair or a bed, only able to walk short distances or very slowly due to pain, and who would have died prematurely because of limited mobility. They can move more freely, play with their children or grandchildren, run, hike, play sports, and have jobs. It is easier for them to be independent. It allowed a man and a woman, in totally different eras, to stand at the altar for their wedding, a child to be a four-year-old, a tightrope walker to resume his profession, a man to become a woodworker so that he could manufacture artificial limbs for fellow amputees, a man who suffered from a fractured hip to walk, an athlete to compete in the Olympics, and countless people to get back to their lives. Rise up and walk is the quintessential miracle.

This relationship of human with mechanical has intrigued writers since the development of the prosthesis. In 1839, Edgar Allan Poe (1809–1849) wrote about Brevet Brigadier General John A. B. C. Smith, a veteran of the Seminole Wars, embittered about the enemy he fought, admired technology of the time, and seemed to be too good to be true. The protagonist was convinced that Smith was hiding something. One morning, on urgent business, he was ushered into Smith's drawing room to only to discover that he was a pile of pieces being assembled by his valet.[59] Herman Melville's (1819–1891) character Captain Ahab stood on a whalebone pegleg, "and, indeed, it seemed small matter for wonder, that for all his pervading, mad recklessness, Ahab did at times give careful heed to the condition of that dead bone; upon which he partly stood."[60] Martin Caidin's (1927–1997) Steve Austin sustained multiple traumatic amputations of both legs and one arm only to be rebuilt stronger and better. This combination was even seen as a possible metaphor for a postmodern polity by Donna Haraway (1944–) in her *A Cyborg Manifesto* published in 1985. She saw the cyborg, the merger of human and mechanical, as a model to escape the dualism that permeated feminist and Marxist thought: "So my cyborg myth is about transgressed boundaries, potent fusions, and dangerous possibilities which progressive people might explore as one part of needed political work."[61]

When Jillian Weise (1981–), a poet and performance artist, describes herself as a cyborg, she is asked if she had read Haraway's *Cyborg Manifesto*. She has. However, she is dismayed that although disabled people like her were the muse for the archetype, she is ultimately omitted from the conversation. Her big decision every night is when to take off her leg, because she is a single woman who lives alone and had been the victim of a stalker. How fast can she run on one leg and a crutch?[62] The popular conception of a person with a prosthesis, whether in a nineteenth-century circular or in the twenty-first-century television story, is daunting to a person, alone, at night, staring down the enormity of a situation they never asked for; when they are enduring pain, when they are struggling through rehabilitation exercises, when, like Ahab, they have to be mindful that their prosthesis, despite everyone's best effort, might catastrophically fail, and when the bravest thing they do is to put themselves together in the morning, like Brigadier General Smith, to get up and face the day.

How we got to this point bothered Robert Duthie, Nuffield Professor of Orthopedic Surgery at Oxford University, who, in 1971, lamented:

> Once again, surgeons are having to solve a problem by actually doing it, e.g., the emporia of Aristotle, which was to acquire knowledge from experience of carrying it out. Fortunately, more attention is being given to the necessary theoretical knowledge, mainly in the field of biomechanics. However, it is necessary to appreciate that surgeons have arrived at this particular point not particularly by logic, but by actually putting in total hip prostheses.[63]

He was bothered that we were learning how to make prosthetics by making prosthetics, a thought process he considered an archaic approach incorrectly attributed to Aristotelian ideology. He advocated a scientific study of biomechanics before designing prosthetics.[64] However, as this account shows that this research was conducted, it was hampered by the difficulty in framing the questions to be answered. The study of biomechanics came from the creation of prostheses, raising questions on how we moved, and the forces sustained by the body. There was no choice but to learn by doing. We did not know what we did not know. In contrast to the academic perspective noted above, Burstein, an engineer, opined: "You can't design knees in an ivory tower."[65] Artificial limbs spurred the study of the process of walking. The artificial hip provided insight into the healing of the bone. Artificial knees spurred the study of the forces sustained by the human body. Ultimately, the most important thing we learned from developing prostheses was the complexity of the basic actions of the human body and the resilience of the human spirit.

NOTES

1. J. Finch et al., "Biomechanical Assessment of Two Artificial Big Toe Restorations from Ancient Egypt and Their Significance to the History of Prosthetics," *J Prosthet Orthot* 24:4 (2012): 181–91.

2. Academy of Orthopaedic Surgeons, *Orthopaedic Appliances Atlas* vol. 2 (Ann Arbor, Mich.: J.W. Edwards, 1960).

3. Hawk, A.J., "How Hemorrhage Control Became Common Sense," J Trauma Acute Care Surg 85 Supplement 1(2018): S13–S17.

4. Phillips, Edward and John Kersey, *The New World of Words: Or, Universal English Dictionary: Containing an Account of the Original or Proper Sense, and Various Significations of All Hard Words Derived from Other Languages . . . Together With a Brief and Plain Explication of All Terms Relating to Any of the Arts And Sciences . . . to Which Is Added, the Interpretation of Proper Names*, 6th ed. (London: Printed for J. Phillips [etc.], 1706).

5. Bell, J., *Engravings of the Bones, Muscles and Joints* (Philadelphia: Anthony Finley, 1818).

6. Birth and death dates unknown.

7. Potts, J. and Lynn, W., "Mr. Potts, on the Means of Supplying the Loss of Amputated Limbs," Med Phys J. 1801, Mar. 5(25): 277–78.

8. Warne, V., "Artificial Leg," *Victorian Review* 34:1(Spring 2008): 29–33.

9. "No 2448 Specification of James Potts: artificial arm and leg, (AD 1800)" London: Great Seal Patent Office (London: George E. Eyre and William Spottiswoode, 1856); and Bigg, H.H., *On artificial limbs, their construction and application* (London: John Churchill, 1855).

10. Baker, R., "The history of gait analysis before the advent of modern computers," *Gait Posture* 26 (2007): 331–42.

11. Robertson, A., *Conversations on Anatomy, Physiology, and Surgery* [vol. 1] (Philadelphia: Towar & Hogan, 1828).

12. Johannsson, E., "Gait Laboratory: Structure and Data Gathering," in Rose, J. and Gamble, J. (ed.), *Human Walking* (Baltimore: Williams & Wilkins, 1994): 139–64; and von Soemmerring, S.T., *Traité d'ostéologie et de syndesmologie, par S.T. Soemmerring suivi d'un traité de la mécanique des organes de la locomotion, par G. et E. Weber, traduit de l'Allemand par A.J.L. Jourdan* (Paris: J.B. Baillière, 1843).

13. Warne (2008).

14. U.S. Patent No. 4,834, "Artificial leg," dated Nov. 4, 1846.

15. "Industrial Exhibition of 1851; American Awards. A List of Awards to United States Contributors at the Great Exhibition of All Nations. I.—Counsel Medicals. II. Prize Medals. III.—Honorable Mention. IV.—Money Award." *New York Times*, Oct. 9, 1851.

16. Holmes, O.W., "The Human Wheel, its Spokes and Felloes," *Atlantic Monthly* (May 1863) [republished by B. Frank Palmer]. Palmer was so pleased with Holmes' article that he subsequently had it published as a pamphlet advertising his artificial limbs.

17. Holmes invented, but didn't patent, a consumer stereoscope in 1859.

18. Holmes (1863).

19. Holmes (1863).

20. Hasegawa, G., *Mending Broken Soldiers* (Carbondale: Southern Illinois University Press, 2012).

21. Marks, A.A., *Marks' Patent Artificial Limbs, with India Rubber Hands and Feet* (New York: William B. Smyth, Job and Card Printer, 1865) and U.S. Patent No. 40,763, "Improvement in Artificial Limbs," Dec. 1, 1863.

22. Marks, G., *A Treatise on Marks' Patent Artificial Limbs with Rubber Hands and Feet* (New York: A. A. Marks, 1888).

23. Marey, Etienne-Jules, *Animal Mechanism: A Treatise on Terrestrial and Aerial Locomotion* (New York: D. Appleton and Co., 1874).

24. Baker (2007).

25. "Muybridge and the Athletes," *The Pennsylvanian* 2:13 (Sept. 28, 1886): 106 [http://hdl.library.upenn.edu/1017/d/archives/20050208003 (accessed Dec. 29, 2022)] and University Archives and Research Center, University of Pennsylvania, *A Guide to the Eadweard Muybridge Collection 1870–1981*, dated Sept. 2008.

26. Marks. G., *Manual of artificial limbs* (New York: A.A. Marks, 1914) and Marks (1888).

27. Marks (1888).

28. Warne (2008).

29. La Vey, D., *The History of Orthopaedics* (Park Ridge: Parthenon Publishing Group, 1990).

30. "Dewey Force Steps on Mine—Loses Right Foot," *Willmar Daily Tribune*, Jan. 1945.

31. "Obituary—Dewey G. Force Jr., 68, psychology professor, dies," *Star Tribune,* June 23, 1989.

32. University of California at Berkeley in National Research Council (U.S.), Committee on Artificial Limbs, *Terminal Research Reports on Artificial Limbs: Report of the Committee on Artificial Limbs of the National Research Council: Covering the Period April 1, 1945 through June 30, 1947* (Washington, D.C.: National Research Council, June 30, 1947): 36–52.

33. Brunnstrom, S., "Anatomical and Physiological Consideration in the Clinical Application of Lower-Extremity Prosthetics," in Academy of Orthopaedic Surgeons, *Orthopaedic Appliances Atlas* vol. 2 (Ann Arbor, Mich.: J. W. Edwards, 1960): 359–82.

34. Sacks, O., "Phantoms," in *The Man Who Mistook His Wife for a Hat* (New York: Summit Books, 1970): 66–76.

35. Wilson, A.B., "Limb Prosthetics Today," Phys Ther. 44:6 (June 1964): 435–69.

36. Desmond, D. and MacLachlan, M., "Psychosocial Issues in the Field of Prosthetics and Orthotics," *J. Prosthet Orthot* 14:1 (March 2002): 19–22.

37. Moore, A. and Bohlman, H., "The Classic: Metal Hip Joint: A Case Report," *Clin Orthop Relat Res*. 453:12(Dec. 2006): 22–24.

38. Moore, A., "The Self-Locking Metal Hip Prosthesis," *J. Bone Surg. Am,* 39A:4 (July 1957): 811–27.

39. Moore (July 1957).

40. Wolff, J., "The Classic: On the Inner Architecture of Bones and Its Importance for Bone Growth," *Clin Orthop Relat Res,* 468:4 (Apr. 2010): 1056–65 and Evans, G., *Stress and Strain in Bones, Their Relation to Fracture and Osteogenesis* (Springfield: Charles C. Thomas, 1957).

41. Moore (July 1957).

42. Campbell, R., and Rothman, R., "Charnley Low Friction Total Hip Replacement," AJR Am J Roentgenol 113:4 (Dec. 1971): 633–41.

43. Walldius, B., "Arthroplasty for the Knee Using an Endoprosthesis: Eight Years' Experience," *Acta Orthop Scand.* 30 (1960): 137–47.

44. Mazas, F.B. and GUEPAR, "Guepar Total Knee Prosthesis," *Clin. Orthop. Relat. Res*, 94 (1973): 211–21.

45. Deburge, A. and GUEPAR, "Guepar Hinge Prosthesis: Complication and Results with Two Years' Follow-up," *Clin. Orthop. Relat. Res*, 120 (1976): 47–53 and Jaffe, W.L., Gross, M.S., and Weinger, E.B., "Guepar hinge knee arthroplasty: A five-year follow-up," *Bull Hosp Jt Dis Orthop Inst*, 42/1 (1982): 17–27.

46. Insall, J.N. and Ranawat, C.S. et al., "A Comparison of Four Models of Total Knee Replacement Prostheses," *J Bone and Joint Surg.* 58A:6 (1976): 754–65.

47. Waugh, T. et al., "Total Knee Replacement," *Clin. Orthop. Relat. Res*, 94 (1973): 196–201.

48. Evans, G., *Stress and Strain in Bones: Their Relation to Fracture and Osteogenesis*, (Springfield: Charles C. Thomas, 1957).

49. Hamilton, L.R., "UCI Total Knee Replacement, A Follow Up Study," *J Bone and Joint Surg. (Am)* 64:5 (June 1982): 740–44.

50. Morrison (1969).

51. Chao, E., Laughman, R., and Stauffer, R., "Biomechanical Gait Evaluation of Pre and Postoperative Total Knee Replacement Patients," *Arch Orthop Traumat Surg* 97 (1980): 309–17.

52. Walldius (1960).

53. Chao (1980).

54. Insall, J., Lachiewicz, F., and Burstein, A., "The Posterior Stabilized: A Modification of the Total Condylar Design. Two to four year clinical experience," *J. Bone Surg. Am* 64:9 (Dec. 1982): 1317–23.

55. Insall, J. et al., "The Total Condylar Prosthesis in Gonarthrosis: Five to Nine Year Follow-up of the First One Hundred Replacements," *J. Bone and Joint Surg (Am)* 65 (1983): 619–28.

56. Orendurff, M. et al., "Gait efficiency using the C-Leg," *J Rehabil Res Dev* 43:2 (Mar-Apr 2006): 239–46.

57. Greenemeir, L., "Blade Runners: Do High-Tech Prostheses Give Runners an Unfair Advantage?" *Scientific American* (Aug. 5, 2016). https://www.scientificamerican.com/article/blade-runners-do-high-tech-prostheses-give-runners-an-unfair-advantage/ (accessed March 9, 2023)

58. Hoellwarth, J. et al., "Osseointegration for Amputees, Current Implants, Techniques, and Future Directions," *JBJS Rev* 8:3 (March 2020): 1–10.

59. Poe, E.A., "The Man That Was Used Up" (1839). https://en.wikisource.org/wiki/The_Man_That_Was_Used_Up (accessed April 15, 2023)

60. Melville, H., *Moby-Dick, or, The Whale* (New York: Harper & Brothers, 1851).
61. Haraway, D., "A Cyborg Manifesto: Science, Technology, and Socialist-Feminism in the Late Twentieth Century," in *Simians, Cyborgs and Women: The Reinvention of Nature* (New York: Routledge, 1991), 149–81.
62. Weise, J., "Common Cyborg," *Granta* (September 24, 2018). https://granta.com/common-cyborg/ (accessed April 23, 2023)
63. Duthie, R.B., "Some observations on present-day hip surgery." *Orthop Clin North Am* 2:1 (Mar. 1971):55–58.
64. Duthie (1971).
65. McGill, D., "Fight for the No. 1 Artificial Knee," *New York Times*, Apr. 25, 1989: D1, D19.

PART III

Pharmaceutical Interventions to the Social World

Chapter 7

Technologies of Repair

Naloxone, Opioid Overdose Prevention, and the Social in the U.S. Southwest

Danielle Kabella

Six days per week mild flows of people return in and out from a quiet room at the end of the hallway at the clinic where they exchange their unsterile needles for up to at least a week's worth of sterile ones. Every-so-often some take interest in direct-service health care through the syringe exchange program as did Flor Garcia,[1] a 44-year-old woman from Albuquerque, who showed up coincidentally on the same day someone dropped out of the out-patient opioid addiction treatment program, for commencing the induction phase of her opioid maintenance therapy. On the Monday that Flor enrolled in the program, stretching her body out from a reclined chair after a combined group treatment of Reiki, acupuncture, and a *limpia* (spiritual cleansing), she along with four other newly enrolled patients and some with friends and family participated in a candid discussion, demonstration, and training on risks and prevention strategies in the event of an overdose, facilitated by a medical apprentice and a physician.

The overdose education was paired with a naloxone prescription for each patient that was part of a targeted proactive strategy to minimize risks of a fatal overdose. Curriculum entailed knowledge about how to rescue someone using naloxone while also navigating the interstitial space of law and health. "When you call 911, be sure to tell them your friend stopped breathing instead of saying they overdosed because they will send cops first and they won't take it as seriously," the instructor said. Attendees were made aware of legal barriers to naloxone like the Good Samaritan Law as well as unmet obligations from legal and medical personnel in upholding their immunity protection.

Patients without their companions in attendance were instructed to enroll close friends and family in their support network and to provide them with naloxone. These strategies are pragmatic on a technical level for a medication that would never be administered by the person receiving it. Bystanders who are familiar with the three forms of naloxone products available—nasal spray, injection, and auto-injection—are encouraged to carry naloxone so that they can be prepared to administer it safely. Having it at home or carrying it on their person not only signals a necessary precaution but a normal one.

Medical anthropologists have considered pharmaceuticals as objects with both medicinal efficacy and interpretative meaning (Mattingly 2000). Thus, who delivers naloxone and who receives it is important especially in the broader context of regulatory failures during an ongoing crisis of opioid overdose and mass incarceration. Naloxone in the hands of family and friends is a transformative milestone in the treatment of addiction because it resituates the relationships between institutions and persons experiencing an overdose. Instead of isolating and incarcerating, we are keeping people in close proximity to each other through its pragmatic approach to achieving life-saving outcomes while learning new ways to care for people who use drugs.

Rising overdose fatalities have brought wider attention to take-home-naloxone as a harm reduction strategy in contemporary public health contexts. Take-home-naloxone is a drug administered by non-medical laypeople to revive someone in the event of an opioid overdose. Take-home-naloxone has become a prominent technological intervention to prevent overdose and is available, with restrictions, in all 50 states as a prescription medication. With a statewide standing order, there is some prescribing authority to co-prescribe and co-distribute under the authority of a licensed physician (with DEA status, even though it's not a controlled substance because there is no potential for abuse) through community-based naloxone programs and syringe exchange programs. There has been considerable debate about its prescription-only status and place of dispensary and the varied challenges they pose to access. There is not a clear geographical or temporal trend in the adoption of access laws and circumstances to regulate vary by state; however, it is notable that New Mexico was the first state to remove legal barriers to take-home-naloxone in 2001 whereas Arizona became the 48th state to pass access laws in 2016 for community distribution.[2] Take-home-naloxone and overdose prevention education were developed as harm-reduction strategies by communities of people who use opioids and advocacy agencies like the Chicago Recovery Alliance in the late 1990s, empowering people who use drugs and their social networks to rescue people who overdose (Dettmer et al. 2001; Maxwell et al. 2006; Campbell 2020). Its distribution has reached, unevenly, populations most at risk for overdose both in proactive, targeted approaches through prescription in opioid treatment programs and prison release programs and in more passive, general access distribution hubs often set up in overdose hotspot zones normally run by grassroots community organizations where people can choose naloxone toward a diversity of goals they have in managing their drug use and on their own terms.

Take-home-naloxone is considered an alternative approach to policy agendas aligned with more punitive measures. Drug control policy has been widely criticized for untying existing bonds between people who use drugs and their social worlds and putting people at greater risk for an overdose. Further, harms inflicted on bodies, families, and communities under punitive drug policies have largely been called into question above all about relatives/peers' lives, the deceased, and relatives/peers' lives who remain detained. If social isolation and stigma make up part of the contextual risk environment (Rhodes 2002) for an overdose, naloxone is one strategy many people could use to restore connection and humanity. Historically there have been disparate drug policy responses that have resulted in carceral outcomes stratified by race and ethnicity (Hansen and Roberts 2012). The demographic profile of the overdose crisis has also shifted over time creating a wider gap in racial disparities for treatment and mortality. Acting both to save lives and support lives, naloxone is being recognized as an alternative approach, and removing its legal barriers to wider access has been regarded as a moment of triumph in the harm reduction movement, drawing its support from many constituencies of varied experiences with the opioid epidemic.

This chapter points to the kind of work take-home-naloxone performs in a world where institutions of abandonment hold out the promise of protection against premature death for people who use drugs. Sometimes affect modalities like fear and animosity are mobilized in these institutions, even as intimate as the family (Clark 2012), to justify the disavowal of life. Yet, social movements have long been sustained by the labor of mothers defending the rights of their children subjected to punitive drug policies (Gilmore 1999). Doing overdose prevention and harm reduction work more broadly requires working under many constraints—enclosure and surveillance, incarceration, the proliferation of stigma and panic, drug prohibition, and coercive legislative impulses—while also mitigating those constraints and keeping people who use drugs safe. In this chapter, rather than framing take-home-naloxone merely as a biological intervention that reduces deaths, I show how, in rearticulating social and familial relationships, take-home-naloxone through its pragmatic approach to reviving life emerges as a step away from normative policy agendas that place emphasis on social arrangements of punishment and isolation by bringing people who use drugs from the fringes to the center of peer and familial networks of care. That is to say, take-home-naloxone is just as social as it is biological—whereby chemical compounds that act on the same opiate receptors in the brain are shared by the person inundated by opiate agonists like morphine or heroin and the person administering the opiate antagonist, naloxone. Naloxone has a stronger affinity to the receptors, knocks them off and replaces them, restoring breathing under the threat of respiratory depression. This interpersonal encounter is key to survival, but it's not free of judicial or political encroachment from decades-old drug policy that isolates people who use drugs from their social worlds through harsh criminal penalties. If it's the depression of breathing that prompts a response from another person, naloxone needs a world otherwise that counteracts the current social arrangements (i.e., isolation, criminalization, homelessness) that keep people at risk for overdose.

In this chapter, I begin with a historical overview of how early take-home-naloxone access laws emerged out of various struggles connected to issues of mass incarceration and premature death led in part by people indirectly experiencing drug harm by biological and fictive kinship—or relationships that take place outside of blood relationships (Nelson 2013), affiliation adding to a rich literature that focuses on the empowering qualities of take-home-naloxone among people who use drugs (Campbell 2020). Then I describe two ethnographic contexts where take-home-naloxone is distributed as 1) a concerted proactive approach in an Opioid Treatment Program (OTP) in New Mexico, which I began this chapter with, and 2) broad distribution efforts in overdose hotspots in Arizona. These sites have existing networks of sociality which makes them ideal places to carry out this study. I argue that take-home-naloxone has a dual function. Its material qualities are used to antagonize chemical interactions in order to rescue people from physiological decline, and it has a social function to aid in creating the social conditions for naloxone to be most effective. Naloxone plays a significant role in stopping an overdose and in the everyday lives of people who use drugs and communities impacted by them. The everyday experience of naloxone may not always be characterized by the event of an overdose, but rather the relationship between bodies and objects.

Take-home-naloxone has shifted the ground on which we stand regarding drugs and the people who use them. To me, take-home-naloxone as a means of standing on different ground means *moving away* from the centrality of the war on drugs, its morally stigmatizing grip, and its social isolation tactics. To be clear, I don't mean to treat lightly the concept "ground" nor evade the fact that I am a scholar who can *move away* from the war on drugs with ease while epitomizing naloxone as an escape route. Part of my methodology is border thinking (Mignolo 2000). Standing on different ground "encompasses the embodiment of epistemological processes emerging from and responding to colonial domination" (Cervantes-Soon and Carrillo, 286).

> A border thinking that originates from coloniality and subalternity rather than from Western thought, it has the potential to offer a new logic and decolonize dominant intellectual thought/knowledge by changing not only the content of discourse but also the locus of enunciation—that is, the place, perspectives and terms through which discourses occur. (Mignolo 2000, 122)

Standing on different ground means meeting people where they are at in their liminal contexts of life and death, agonized and antagonized, isolation and connection, pain and pleasure, habit and disease, and so on; and others not so easily categorized or resisting altogether. In this chapter, I showcase the emergence of take-home-naloxone from the places and people that encounter its objects to capture new ideas about what it means to care for people who use drugs.

Similarly, part of my ethnographic approach and theory-building is recognizing the ground on which *I* stand or what feminist scholars call standpoint theory (Collins 1997). I bring several situated, partial perspectives to bear on this inquiry about overdose, naloxone, and drug war politics as refracted through my own professional-personal positionality as a queer, chicanx, harm reductionist with experience navigating the world at varied middle to bottom levels of the social hierarchy. For many the bottom brings a whole lot of structural injustices—poverty, trauma, drugs, etc. For me, as someone who has some ground to stand on in the matter, drug use and drug war–related family separation felt readily available to me in terms of years of professional experience, lived experience, and expertise. My parents were people who used drugs, and while it was chaotic and destabilizing at times, I became intuitive to the stigmatizing, alienating, and racializing drug policies that intensified our precarity. From this perspective, I recognize that people detained and deceased to drugs are people embedded in families and communities. I take seriously the role of kinship (biological and fictive) in the development of human rights justice for people who use drugs including take-home-naloxone and the emergent form it takes on as a technology of repair. I will describe in further detail in the cases that follow.

NEW MEXICO DRUG REFORM, NALOXONE ACCESS, AND HUMAN RIGHTS 2001

By March 1999, the northern rural town of Espanola, New Mexico, gained national attention as a place of crisis in overdose fatalities, adopting the nickname "overdose capital of the world." In 2001, New Mexico became the first state to remove legal barriers to the distribution of take-home-naloxone. The sanctioning experiment of take-home-naloxone makes sense considering rising overdose rates in New Mexico (a place in overdose crisis) and might at first seem like the only logical place to advance drug reform given the political authority the state had at the time to publicly denounce the war on drugs for its failure to stem drug use. Yet, efforts that belie drug reform transcend the boundaries of the state's authority. And saving lives was not the outcome of naloxone's technological innovation alone. It was neither one institution that willed take-home-naloxone into existence. Rather, sanctioning take-home-naloxone in New Mexico was part of a larger reform project that emerged from a set of struggles connected to national trends of mass incarceration, overdose fatalities, drug-related HIV/HCV deaths, and the harm reduction movement that transgressed state (and national) boundaries.

The story of naloxone is often told from the perspective of Dan Bigg, Sarz Maxwell, and Karen Stanczykiewicz and other brave harm reductionists at the Chicago Recovery Alliance (CRA) who in the 1990s got ahead of the opioid epidemic in Chicago by putting naloxone directly into the hands of people who use drugs before it was made legal (Maxwell et al. 2006; Campbell 2020). Nancy Campbell (2020) has done a compelling study that associates this narrative with the empowerment of people who use drugs in having access to life-saving medicine and resources to take care of themselves and each other. CRA's experiment with naloxone no doubt had an impact on wider access to naloxone in New Mexico and the rest of the country. However, the perspective I offer here is a moment in history when New Mexico, as the first state to do so, adopted take-home-naloxone into law. A close look at the data brought me to varied stories of activism associated with experiences of drug harm through kinship affiliation and stories of families impacted by the war on drugs. These stories helped set in motion naloxone access laws contained in Republican governor Gary Johnson's "overhaul" package profuse with "leading-edge drug reform measures in New Mexico, that, bottom-line, would reduce the harm that drugs create on our society."[3]

On August 1, 2000, Governor Johnson was invited to speak about local drug reform efforts along with Reverend Jesse Jackson and other public figures at the University of Pennsylvania's Annenberg Center for a national drug policy forum in a Shadow Convention event attended by more than a thousand people. The focus of the event was two-fold: drug-related public health harms like the spread of AIDS, HIV, and HCV, and overdose deaths and the rise of mass incarceration. Families, wearing shirts with photos of deceased and incarcerated relatives, accustomed to reclaiming the fragments of their shattered lives in the dark (and in shame) were fearlessly leading emotional ceremonies, turning their private grief into public memorials of people jailed on mandatory minimums and lives lost to failed public health policies. Youth performed songs and poems in remembrance of parents incarcerated. Children gave testimony about losing parents to drug-related AIDS and hepatitis C, turning their deaths into advocacy for syringe exchange programs[4] and harm reduction measures. Ethan Nadelmann, the director of the Drug Policy Alliance (then the Lindesmith Center and Drug Policy Foundation) and a convener of the Shadow Conventions, declared this "the biggest day in the young history of the drug policy" and the beginning of a "new anti-war movement . . . a movement to end the war on drugs, a movement that may prevent a wider war in another country, a movement that calls for drug policies based upon common sense, science, public health, and human rights" (US Newswire 2000).

In a more concerted effort to gain support for his overall drug reform package (including the pioneering legislation for naloxone) from lawmakers back home in New Mexico, Johnson met with the grassroots human rights organization New York Mothers of the Disappeared on July 17, 2001 (Olaechea 2001, B3). During their visit, the mothers shared their personal experiences with the governor and participated in a joint press conference at a local hotel drawing attention to the social harm that long sentences for non-violent drug offenses have on families and their disproportionate effects on African American and Hispanic communities. New Mexico was one of three stops they made in their tour of the Southwest in their advocacy efforts. The others were cities in Texas including Tulia, which is famously known for a drug sting operation that was called into question after the detective leading the operation that targeted an African American community made unfounded claims and deceitful testimony. Race and drugs have a long history in the U.S., and this angle of harm reduction opened the door to racial injustice. The mothers participated in the "Never Again" rally commemorating the 2-year anniversary of the controversial sting before joining the NAACP Forum in Amarillo on topics of race and the drug war. It was the complaints that bolstered a public health approach to substance use that the governor absorbed into his reform package. Nevertheless, the mutual effort attracted the mothers to the reform package to focus on decriminalization and harm reduction. Yet, the mothers' advocacy around drug harm turned it into a human rights campaign that brought attention to incarceration, race, and defending that lives are not expendable.

The New York Mothers of the Disappeared was a group of mothers who had been formerly incarcerated, or their relatives were in prison serving long sentences for low-level drug crimes. The group modeled themselves after the Mothers of the Disappeared, the women who marched weekly at the Plaza de Mayo in Argentina to draw attention to loved ones killed by military troops, by organizing vigils to draw attention to the issue (Arditti 1999; Smith 2016). Like in post-conflict Argentina, the women who sought state restitution for their children, the New York Mothers of the Disappeared were more than drug reform activists, they were also fighting repression and defending human rights. Through public engagement with policy officials and educational workshops, New York Mothers of the Disappeared coordinated advocacy efforts to expose human rights violations from the U.S. drug war and the consequential social harm effects of incarceration on families. Like the Disappeared of Argentina, drug offenders (and users) in the U.S. live in social worlds of kinship ties and families—they are sons, daughters, grandchildren, cousins, uncles, aunts, friends, peers, and neighbors. Memorializing their legacies came at a time when the drug war harms needed to be personified.

Johnson's strategy to "put a face" to the drug war (and the victims targeted for policy reform) was a strategy from the New York Mothers of the Disappeared's playbook primarily focused on abolishing the 1971 Rockefeller laws but extending their activism to policies that had life-altering consequences for people who used drugs. To law enforcement, child welfare agents, and even the state, people who used drugs were uniformly drug-criminal subversives and a threat to national security—public enemy number one. Stripped of any social identity as wards of the state, they were, at worst, as nonexistent as those of the disappeared, numbers in a growing prison population, and faceless statistics in overdose counts, at best. To their mothers and their relatives, they were whole humans; knowing the depth of their vibrant social identities, at the core, they were ultimately someone's relative. In a historical alliance between the Argentina Mothers and the New York Mothers, Almeya, an Argentine mother, expressed her solidarity efforts across nations: "Their children and relatives are also desaparecidos, unjustly taken away from family and society for years on end. We are with them demanding the abolition of the unfair Rockefeller laws" (Kunstler Fund 2004).

Like the Rockefeller laws in 1971 of mandatory minimums and the New York–based group Mothers of the Disappeared who saw their suffering as part of a world system, finding inspiration from the mothers who confronted the military on the basis of moral authority was empowering. This mother-to-mother coalition saw an injustice of disappearing their children in a political system of repression (activism in Argentina in the 1980s) or extended prison sentences for non-violent drug offenses (activism in the U.S. in the 1990s), both fighting repression and for human rights from a place of intimacy and care. This laid down a path for naloxone, and harm reduction measures to unfold to the public. These were networks that mobilized naloxone access laws into existence that happened nationally and internationally (as far as Argentina) to bring attention to state repression from the organizing power of maternal communities.

Using the decriminalization narrative echoed across the globe, Johnson insisted that when police arrive at the scene of overdose, people will first be revived by trying to save their life with naloxone (which was used exclusively in emergency room settings at first) instead of preparing for an arrest. This was part of Johnson's overall philosophy on drug reform, who in the early 2000s was a strong proponent against the drug war in politics at the time.

The access laws presented a new challenge to non-medical laypeople to administer it and who might be held accountable for criminal and/or civil liability. The passage of the Good Samaritan Law came in 2008 to protect immunity. This altered liability law for police and others to administer Narcan without fear of civil suits. Although imperfect, this technology was a first attempt at changing the direct relationship between law enforcement and health. What is important is that it challenged drug laws that regulated who can dispense/administer aid as well as who can be recipients of aid in the event of an overdose. This was the first step in decriminalization, or of unsettling the 30 years of draconian drug laws for the first time. The struggle began from lived experience, and drug policy was first targeted by family and peers ushering in the possibility for more public health and harm reduction approaches for overdose prevention.

OVERDOSE EDUCATION AND NALOXONE TRAINING, NEW MEXICO, 2013

After twenty-two years of take-home-naloxone in New Mexico, several experiments have emerged around how best to equip people most at risk for an overdose with this lifesaving drug. In 2017, New Mexico mandated that take-home-naloxone and overdose education be supplemented in Opioid Treatment Programs and Prison Release programs (Katzman et al. 2020). One of the earliest programs to implement this policy, before it was mandated by law and as a targeted harm reduction strategy, was the small family medical clinic Casa de Salud. Casa de Salud is a vital access point for harm reduction and innovative drug recovery services in New Mexico offering a spectrum of services as described in the opening vignette: syringe services, Medication-Assisted Treatment (MAT), alternative healing practices, and targeted naloxone education and distribution. In the process of starting the low-cost family medical clinic in a Spanish-speaking, mixed immigration, low-income environment, serving people with little or no insurance in a neighborhood of Albuquerque, one of the founding physicians remembers that "working in the South Valley, it was just in our face every day, particularly with heroin, it just kind of came raging at us as an issue to address." Turning to a harm reduction approach, they started a needle exchange program funded by the Department of Health in 2005 which also served as an innovative way to pay for the clinic while keeping prices fair for self-pay along with insurance. A culturally sensitive treatment component was built out of a needle exchange program which had a take-home-naloxone training and drug curriculum built into it performed by healing practitioners, medical apprentices, and physicians in a group setting as part of their induction phase for medically assisted therapy in the treatment of opioid addiction.

Culturally competent care in the context of harm reduction is unique in and of itself—the vision for the clinic from the beginning was to integrate Western medicine with alternative medicine through a partnership between physicians and a local healing collective consisting of *curanderas* (traditional healers) designed to accommodate the clientele in a setting where service entry is most common in patients from very diverse racial, socioeconomic, and family backgrounds. The approach overall is peripheral to the hegemony of abstinence-based addiction therapeutics and is an example of health initiatives from grassroots organizations. Take-home-naloxone emerged within this coordination of care which emphasized a holistic approach (e.g., cultural, psycho-social, spiritual) rather than a reductionist view of the body (e.g., biological) through emphasizing relationships not only with the self but also with others. Whereas under the authority of Western medicine, bodies are processed in standardized and routine ways, at the clinic patients were treated as whole beings with strategies to try to balance and integrate these dimensions into the process of recovery. Nonetheless, naloxone at the clinic emerged within already existing social, economic, and technical relations and was set up as one strategy to reduce drug-related harms in culturally competent, non-judgmental ways.

When I visited the clinic in the summer of 2013, take-home-naloxone was used as a proactive strategy to minimize risks of an overdose. Two doses of take-home-naloxone were prescribed along with overdose education and training provided to each patient in the Opioid Treatment Program. The program was unique in that patients were required[5] to attend four healing circles with healing practitioners trained in Western, Eastern, and Traditional medicine, whereas a cohort would collectively spend two hours learning about addiction, harm reduction services, overdose education and naloxone training as well as receive combined healing modalities—Reiki, acupuncture, and *limpia* (spiritual cleansing)—in a single session with time reserved at the end to debrief as a group. The healing circles departed from single-transactional exchanges that have no sense of sociality. Patients described the impact it had on them. One patient explained how the healers helped improve the relationship she had with herself: "I think they kind of remind you it's ok to love yourself and be gentle with yourself. It's ok. Do that. And it's okay." Another described the relationship with her family had improved since sharing the knowledge; "they give you these little fliers that have good sayings, and I always put them on the refrigerator at my dad's, and he used to read them. I put them there because he used to judge people [who use drugs]." In this sense, naloxone wasn't just handed out to the patients, it was engulfed in the entire experience of coordinated companionate care focused around reducing biological death and socializing the impact of the harms and ways to reduce them to the self and others, recasting people who use drugs as humans with needs for compassion and understanding.

Take-home-naloxone was entangled with practices of care at the clinic in contradictory ways: people in recovery may develop insobriety and yet they need direct connection. For instance, during the naloxone training, patients collaboratively engaged in a curriculum developed in a way that the ideas of individuals would accumulate into a collective understanding of how to prepare and respond in the event of an overdose and subsequently receive a refillable prescription for two doses of naloxone to be shared with close friends and family. The effects of naloxone were explained to patients and their peers and families.

To show how take-home-naloxone rearticulates peer and familial relationships, it's important to understand how it works. When someone's system is inundated with opioids their breathing begins to shallow and they are incapable of restoring normal breathing on their own. This prompts a response from another person, preferably someone trained in recognizing the signs of an overdose—slowed breathing, pale skin, unconsciousness, etc.—and to confirm it most effectively with a sternum rub. If the person doesn't respond, this prompts the person to administer naloxone: intramuscular or nasally. When naloxone is in the body, it acts on the same opioid receptors and restores breathing within 2 to 5 minutes by knocking off the opioids from the receptors and replacing them with naloxone and blocking the effects of remaining opioids. The person immediately goes into symptomatic withdrawal from the drug. This agonist-antagonist relationship at the level of the brain models the relationship needed for care—the agonist (a body with opioids), the antagonist (naloxone), and someone to administer it.

The demonstration made clear that one of the best indicators of surviving a drug overdose is if you are in direct line of sight of another human being. While the person inundated with opioids is being rescued from physiological decline before succumbing to a fatal overdose, another person is inserting a needle in the upper arm muscle or a nozzle tip in the nostril and plunging the medication into their body. The simulated overdose in the demonstration put naloxone's dual function into sharp focus. First, the physiological function, in response to an overdose, of the chemical compounds of opiate antagonists (naloxone) having a stronger affinity to the same opiate receptors in the brain than heroin or morphine (agonist opiates) knocking them off, replacing them, and blocking the effects of the remaining heroin. Second, the formulation of the product—vial and syringe or nasal spray—requires someone other than the person receiving the medication to administer it. In the context of an overdose, they must recognize the physiological signs which prompts an immediate response. This coordination of overdose care with family and friends fulfilled a proactive role in stopping an overdose. But most importantly, the care that surrounded the demonstration—socializing people to the phenomenon of an overdose through the treatment of it—suggests naloxone not only plays a significant role in preventing overdose but in the everyday lives of people who use drugs and communities impacted by drugs. The interactions between objects and bodies aid in the creation of space in which fewer deaths may occur and the proliferation of collective strategies to keep people safe.

The effects measure up both with and beyond naloxone's potent pharmaceutical properties. One of opioids' friendly foes is naloxone, first to quickly attack by antagonizing opioid receptors at the brain then to protect with greater binding affinity, reversing heroin's effects of respiratory failure and returning to the lungs some of the breath that was lost. Like its alchemy, two people are linked by antagonized chemical bonds putting into sharp focus take-home-naloxone's dual function. A material bond intended for the body to evade biological death and scaled up to reclaim the living from the violence of isolation and social death. In rearticulating the social, naloxone takes on an emergent form as a technology of repair (Smith 2017). It is this socio-material phenomenon that could wrestle away some of these totalizing notions of the "addict," drawing attention to new encounters and the stories told around them.

The benefit of take-home-naloxone hinges synchronously on its pharmaceutical effects and social elements. Like in the demonstration at the clinic I began this chapter with how naloxone channels attention to the people and social networks it implicates across varied experiences of advocacy, everyday modes of survival, treatment, education and distribution, and administration. Its place between the clinic and home is significant because home constitutes a realm of intimate social ties with family (given and chosen), peers, and partners, and taking it there allows the technology to take on an emergent form as a technology of repair. Home is also the most common place where drug overdose occurs (Sporer 1999). Notably, take-home-naloxone implicates family, peers, and partners in new ways and their active roles open possibilities to reimagine the terms of the body in the form of care, to redraw the boundaries of drug use across a spectrum of strategies for safe use, managed use, or abstinence as well as transforming the space of recovery where bodies, care, and managed drug use can coexist in the home. In this section I attempted to show how take-home-naloxone is used in a treatment setting, a setting which already emphasizes social ties and family/peer support. The act of giving someone naloxone at home is profound because it is where active roles for family and friends begin to unfold with the potential to shift the way we care for people who use drugs while considering first the preservation of human life above all else.

SOMATIC EXPERTISE AND NALOXONE DISTRIBUTION, PHOENIX, ARIZONA, 2022

There are many strategies to distribute naloxone. Unlike the proactive naloxone prescription at the clinic described above, naloxone distribution is also a passive effort where, through a statewide standing prescription order, codistribution can take place by a harm reduction organization or a syringe exchange program. This can take place in a variety of ways. I focus in this section on street-based outreach services where harm reduction workers go to a designated overdose hotspot for a consistent scheduled day and time of the week, where they provide several safe-use supplies including naloxone. No one is required or mandated to take naloxone, but it is available upon request, and they can take as many as they need. In these spaces, people will take naloxone either for themselves or people they know or who they are in proximity to. For transient communities, this could be people in a shared encampment.

Fifteen years after take-home-naloxone was sanctioned in New Mexico, legislation was passed in Arizona in 2016; in 2018 the Good Samaritan Law was passed; and finally in 2021 syringe exchange services were decriminalized. Before that naloxone was outlawed in Arizona, forcing distribution networks underground. One such organization was Sonoran Prevention Works (SPW) to offer harm reduction services in Arizona. SPW was founded by and for people who use drugs with the intention that people have the tools, knowledge, and community to be safe and healthy. Since 2011 they have been distributing sterile syringes, initially via bicycle delivery, at large monthly events in downtown Phoenix. Although overdose was on the rise in 2014, take-home-naloxone was banned, yet with the help of other organizations they took their operations underground until 2016 when Arizona became the 48th state to sanction take-home-naloxone access via a standing order. Quickly ramping up their efforts, they created statewide Overdose Education and Naloxone Distribution extending knowledge and naloxone access across Arizona.

During fieldwork, I volunteered with SPW in the summer of 2022 doing street-based outreach where I was trained on administering rapid HIV/ HCV testing and carried out this work along with bringing safe-use supplies including naloxone to predominantly unsheltered communities, especially those who are at risk for contracting hepatitis C and/or HIV, in Tempe, Arizona. SPW is Arizona's statewide harm reduction and largest Naloxone lay distributor in the United States. In this section, I show how in zones of abandonment, naloxone is distributed through coordinated efforts of peer support and draws people into public spaces.

Up until recently before the encampment sweeps in the city of Tempe, Tuesday evenings you could find me at a local park in Tempe, only one mile from Arizona State University. Between the evening hours of 4 and 6 pm, the park is lively with people occupying the grassland to its fullest extent. As part of a larger outreach operation organized by organizations that provide support for the unhoused, the public park is transformed into a makeshift free market for transient unhoused neighbors. The perimeter of the park is lined with collectives and grassroots organizations offering services anywhere from free vaccinations for pets, hot meals, used and unused clothing, government-subsidized cell phone services, basic first aid, and nonperishable foods. When the truck pulls up with tents and donated clothing, people flock to the center to sort through the boxes of clothing and personal hygiene products. Carrying a bag of clothing, booties to protect their dogs' feet from the scorching asphalt in Arizona's unforgiving summer heat, and rushing to the food lines that rotate a hot meal from a local restaurant nearby. In our spot under a shaded tree, we offer HIV and hepatitis C testing in exchange for a monthly bus pass as well as hand out safe-use and safe-sex supplies, fentanyl test strips, and naloxone. Setting up our table, only a few meters from the nearest bus stop where the Orbit, or the university commuter and the Metro-wide bus systems, drops off waves of people who cooperatively comply to a sense of order in a seemingly chaotic experience. It can be quite overwhelming as people approach you for several needs. Yet we build a sense of community as we begin to recognize the faces or needs and those of service informing each other of services available. This mutual aid effort was unfortunately cut short due to a growing trend in encampment sweeps that hit hard in the city, targeting the unhoused and forcing organizations to jump through permit hoops to congregate. People often talk of the growing high-rises in Tempe to meet the housing needs of incoming university students and the growing development and gentrification that surrounds it. The sweeps support development efforts for luxury apartments for incoming students.

This transient group is commuting longer distances with the city of Tempe's recent crackdown, evicting people from encampments at the riverbanks on Tempe Town Lake to the bridges at the overpass. Some walked or took a bicycle. Rushing to form a line, most were there for a bus pass as compensation for HIV and hepatitis C rapid tests. Others needed supplies for safe use and safe sex.

Negotiating the park space with residents and the health needs of unsheltered neighbors facing displacement upon eviction of the encampments and extreme heat makes homelessness in Phoenix notably brutal. Still for those who themselves or have friends who need naloxone, approach me with grace.

A place that brings us both together for a fleeting two hours one day a week. I have something that draws them to my table—naloxone—so that they can go back to encampments and use it on their neighbors.

It is an intimate encounter to take someone's hand in yours and extract blood from it. People open up to me and demonstrate courage to ask questions and to even be critical. This informs my strategy for counseling them on disease containment and management that requires gaining "strategic knowledge," which is essentially the practice of research. Appadurai, an American Indian anthropologist, talks about this notion of the "right to research" as a special kind of right that is vital for survival and the exercise of citizenship (2006). A "right to research" entails broadening the research enterprise from a highly specialized field exclusive to "experts" to a more elementary and universal capacity for research that is carried out by ordinary people through a process of "documentation as intervention" (Appadurai 2006, 176). The right to know something that is previously unknown is an act of informed citizenship. People can use knowledge to advocate for themselves and their communities by attending to their own life circumstances through systematically gathering basic information. To collectively gain strategic knowledge gives context to where they are living, how they are accessing food, water, sanitary facilities, and the other basic necessities. Their access to safe-use supplies expands their options to keep them safe and healthy through harm reduction practices like not sharing or reusing their works and using safe-sex supplies like condoms. From there I can get information about their susceptibility to disease because of greater chances of exposure and lack of resources and it helps me guide the educational portion of the assessment. My inquiry depends: "Do you know how HIV and Hep C are contracted?" or "Have you recently used naloxone and how many overdose reversals did you perform?" The questions are guideposts for educational guidance that challenges me to explain all of this in a way that is non-stigmatizing and informative and quick because a growing line of about fifteen people forms for testing. Yet, in the fifteen minutes of our encounter they ask bold questions and challenge their own or even my perspective. Most notably we develop a relationship that is authentic and opens the door to learning and advocating for what they need.

If naloxone has been ushered in to preserve bare life, what somatic ethics has it brought to these aspects? I show how new forms of expertise emerge to support an ethics of care and support and guidance and consultation in these outreach encounters. Somatic expertise (Rose 2007, 6) consists of harm reduction outreach workers who support and care and guide and counsel people who use drugs safely through checking of contaminated drugs, testing for HIV/HCV, using naloxone, and not using alone.

CONCLUSION

I conducted a study that looked at three contexts where naloxone emerges as a heterogenous technology. I found that efforts were more than the outcome of pharmaceutical effects acting on the biological body and extend to social worlds that emerge otherwise. The social elements of overdose management via naloxone put into sharp focus that naloxone is most effective when it is part of coordinated care efforts that prioritize social, peer, and familial relationships. This is significant because the recognition of ineffective drug policies from the failed war on drugs are being called into question. Punitive measures can no longer resolve drug use and in fact new definitions of drug use, recovery, and methods to reduce risks both to the biological and social body are needed.

Take-home-naloxone has shifted the ground on which we stand regarding drugs and the people who use them. To me, take-home-naloxone as a means of standing on different ground means *moving away* from the centrality of the war on drugs, its morally stigmatizing grip, and its social isolation tactics. The ground, however, is not neutral and for some more than others take-home-naloxone has "unmet obligations" (Lopez et al. 2022); it functions primarily as "palliative governance" reducing the extremely marginalized to biological bare life (DiMario 2022) or as a "technology of whiteness" as white racial rescue (Hansen et al. 2023). These are valid cautions. Naloxone isn't capable of *ending* the Drug War or its racializing grip and its drug enforcement, child welfare, and mass-incarceration projects. These are many of the social harm effects that are too large to ignore, indeed. How do we begin to acknowledge the accumulated losses of incarceration, death, child separation from the Drug War while putting pressure on those responsible (i.e., pharmaceutical companies profiting off deaths of many now making reparations by paying off lawsuits)? We can hold naloxone in critique's line of sight while putting forward possibilities for what might be to gain: For whom? And for what purposes?

The outcomes of this research have provided insight into an overlooked aspect of the social history of naloxone. By contextualizing naloxone access laws, this research fills a gap in the literature by focusing on the role of family/kinship in policy reform and complements naloxone's history after it was emancipated by people who use drugs and advocates, the most well known by Dan Biggs in the Chicago Recovery Alliance and their important grassroots work in emancipating the technology from emergency medicine (Campbell 2020). Situated in New Mexico and Arizona, we see a partial history and a set of events that brought widespread access. Mothers defending the rights of their sons, daughters, and relatives who "disappeared" to a system of repression and death by holding public vigils to memorialize lives lost to drugs and drug-related harms as well as lives who remain detained under racialized drug policies. Seen in this context, the discourse of kinship (fictive and biological) became a translational object between political activism and social benefits of a medically assisted intervention of overdose as part of a larger strategy to demand state accountability and social policy reform in response to a failing drug war. Further, after several years with the experiment of sanctioned naloxone are innovative experiments that challenge further the biological basis for overdose prevention and show its wider implications in considering the whole body including the social.

In terms of rearticulating the social, naloxone's pharmaceutical effects are shaped by and shape social interaction, and even more potent is the dynamic entanglements of caring practices and relationships that naloxone works to affirm—the humanity of people who use drugs as people who are ultimately embedded in social and familial networks—and that these very networks optimize naloxone's effectiveness.

Increasingly, however, across the nation and internationally, from emergency medicine and science to social policy and public health, naloxone-practices to keep people who use drugs alive has been explicated and managed through the manipulation of opposing chemicals at the site of the receptor. At this moment, the effectiveness of the medication is afforded by the design of the product—prepackaged nasal spray and syringe and vial—which depend on the presence of another human being who is knowledgeable about slowed or stopped breathing, among other signs, and administering the drug. This is an investment that constitutes a kind of relationship that is not required in the same way as other overdose prevention strategies.

For example, advocacy initiatives like "don't use alone" hotlines and public health interventions like safe injection sites are premised on the idea that social relationships and larger social networks are vital for people who use drugs. They assume drug use is unsafe when done in isolation. Other strategies like fentanyl test strips that test for fentanyl in the drug supply can be administered by a single person but are distributed in harm reduction organizations through street outreach. Yet naloxone requires a particular dynamic. It is distributed to family and friends and social networks that are most crossed by people who use drugs, embedding them into a network of care that challenges the drug war logics of isolation, incarceration, and alienation.

ACKNOWLEDGEMENTS

Thank you to all the people who participated in this study. This research was supported by Arizona State University's Dissertation Completion Fellowship and an NIH/NIDA-funded Postdoctoral Training Fellowship in Tobacco Control (T32DA057216).

NOTES

1. Flor Garcia, interview with author, November 2013. During the research, the author asked individuals to indicate whether they would like their full legal name used in publications. Given the type of stigma associated with drug use in the U.S., careful use of names and respect for the wishes of individuals was maintained by the author.

2. On March 29, 2023, Narcan nasal spray became the first U.S. FDA approved over-the-counter naloxone product for use without a prescription. It is being sold directly to consumers in places like drug stores, convenience stores, grocery stores, gas stations, and online.

3. Johnson said in an interview with *Nightline* host Ted Koppel (Terrell 2001).

4. Possessing syringes was illegal in most states in 2001 and still is in some states.

5. Casa de Salud's treatment policies have changed since my fieldwork. There are no longer conditions for treatment and alternative healing is voluntary.

REFERENCES

Ahmad, F.B., L.M. Rossen, and P. Sutton. 2021. "Provisional drug overdose death counts." U.S. Department of Health and Human Services, National Center for Health Statistics. https://www.cdc.gov/nchs/nvss/vsrr/drug-overdose-data.htm

Arditti, R. 1999. *Searching for Life: The Grandmothers of the Plaza de Mayo and the Disappeared Children of Argentina*. Berkeley: University of California Press.

Campbell, Nancy D. 2020. *OD: Naloxone and the Politics of Overdose*. MIT Press.

Cervantes-Soon, Claudia G. and Juan F. Carrillo. "Toward a pedagogy of border thinking: Building on Latin@ students' subaltern knowledge." *The High School Journal* 99, no. 4 (2016): 282–301.

Clark, Claire D. "Tough love: A brief cultural history of the addiction intervention." *History of Psychology* 15, no. 3 (2012): 233.

Collins, Patricia Hill. "'Standpoint Theory Revisited': Where's the Power?" *Signs: Journal of Women in Culture and Society* 22, no. 2 (1997).

Dettmer, Kerstin, Bill Saunders, and John Strang. "Take home naloxone and the prevention of deaths from opiate overdose: two pilot schemes." *BMJ* 322, no. 7291 (2001): 895–896.

DiMario, Anthony. "To Punish, Parent, or Palliate: Governing Urban Poverty through Institutional Failure." *American Sociological Review* 87, no. 5 (2022): 860–888.

Farrugia, Adrian, Suzanne Fraser, and Robyn Dwyer. "Assembling the social and political dimensions of take-home naloxone." *Contemporary Drug Problems* 44, no. 3 (2017): 163–175.

Faulkner-Gurstein, Rachel. "The social logic of naloxone: Peer administration, harm reduction, and the transformation of social policy." *Social Science & Medicine* 180 (2017): 20–27.

Gilmore, Ruth Wilson. "You have dislodged a boulder: Mothers and prisoners in the post Keynesian California landscape." *Transforming Anthropology* 8, no. 1–2 (1999): 12–38.

Hansen, Helena, Jules Netherland, and David Herzberg. 2023. *Whiteout: How Racial Capitalism Changed the Color of Opioids in America*. University of California Press.

Katzman, Joanna G., Mikiko Y. Takeda, Nina Greenberg, Monica Moya Balasch, Amal Alchbli, William G. Katzman, Julie G. Salvador, and Snehal R. Bhatt. "Association of take-home naloxone and opioid overdose reversals performed by patients in an opioid treatment program." *JAMA Network Open* 3, no. 2 (2020): e200117.

Kunstler Fund. "Moms add muscle to reform drug laws." April 15, 2004. http://www.kunstler.org/madres2.html

Kunstler Fund. "Rockefeller Drug Laws Vigils." Accessed January 26, 2023. http://kunstler.org/projects.html

Lopez, A.M., M. Thomann, Z. Dhatt, J. Ferrera, M. Al-Nassir, M. Ambrose, and S. Sullivan. 2022. "Understanding racial inequities in the implementation of harm reduction initiatives." *American Journal of Public Health* 112(S2): S173–S181.

Mattingly, Cheryl, and Linda C. Garro, eds. Narrative and the cultural construction of illness and healing. University of California Press, 2000.

Maxwell, S., D. Bigg, K. Stanczykiewicz, and S. Carlberg-Racich. 2006. "Prescribing naloxone to actively injecting heroin users: A program to reduce heroin overdose deaths." *J Addict Dis.* 25(3): 89–96. doi: 10.1300/J069v25n03_11. PMID: 16956873.

McDonald, Rebecca, Nancy D. Campbell, and John Strang. "Twenty years of take-home naloxone for the prevention of overdose deaths from heroin and other opioids—conception and maturation." *Drug and Alcohol Dependence* 178 (2017): 176–187.

Mignolo, W. (2000). *Local histories/global designs: Coloniality, subaltern knowledges, and border thinking*. Princeton, NJ: Princeton University Press.

Nelson, Margaret K. "Fictive kin, families we choose, and voluntary kin: What does the discourse tell us?" *Journal of Family Theory & Review* 5, no. 4 (2013): 259–281.

Niles, J.K., J. Gudin, J. Radcliff, and H.W. Kaufman. "The opioid epidemic within the COVID-19 pandemic: Drug testing in 2020." *Population Health Management* 24 (S1) (2021). doi: 10.1089/pop.2020.0230. 43-S-75.

Olaechea, Alma. "Conference Highlights Rehabilitation of Addicts in Prison." *Albuquerque Journal*, July 18, 2001, B3.

Rhodes, Tim. "The 'risk environment': A framework for understanding and reducing drug-related harm." *International Journal of Drug Policy* 13, no. 2 (2002): 85–94.

"Senate OKs overdose-antidote bill." *Santa Fe New Mexican* (New Mexico). March 12, 2001.

"Shadow Convention Hosts Most Important Drug Policy Forum Ever Held at a National Political Convention." U.S. Newswire. August 1, 2000. https://

advance-lexis-com.ezproxy1.lib.asu.edu/api/document?collection=news&id=urn:contentItem:40W3-X9Y0-0007-24RN-00000-00&context=1516831.

Smith, Lindsay Adams. "Identifying democracy: Citizenship, DNA, and identity in postdictatorship Argentina." *Science, Technology, & Human Values* 41, no. 6 (2016): 1037–1062.

Smith, Lindsay A. "The missing, the martyred and the disappeared: Global networks, technical intensification and the end of human rights genetics." *Social Studies of Science* 47, no. 3 (2017): 398–416.

Sporer, Karl A. "Acute heroin overdose." *Annals of Internal Medicine* 130, no. 7 (1999): 584–590.

Strang, John, Shane Darke, Wayne Hall, Michael Farrell, and Robert Ali. "Heroin overdose: The case for take-home naloxone." *BMJ* 312, no. 7044 (1996): 1435–1436. https://advance-lexis com.ezproxy1.lib.asu.edu/api/document?collection=news&id=urn:contentIem:42JJ-PS90-0093-C0DB-00000-00&context=1516831. https://drugpolicy.org/news/2000/07/unprecedented-momentum-builds-against-americasdrug-war-more-1000-prepare-gather-shadow-

Terrell, Steve. "Johnson takes drug proposals to 'Nightline.'" *Santa Fe New Mexican* (New Mexico). January 30, 2001. https://advance-lexis-com.ezproxy1.lib.asu.edu/api/document?collection=news&id=urn:contentItem:427T-5DD0-0093-C388-00000-00&context=1516831.

Chapter 8

Abilify MyCite and the Social Control of Digital Pills

Kathryn Burrows

The assertion of social control over individuals with known medical conditions has been promulgated since the dawn of germ theory in the mid-nineteenth century (Newton 2020). As soon as it was realized that people could give or transmit disease to other people, and that illness wasn't caused by supernatural forces (Newton 2020), the public, and public officials, have tried to assert control over those people who were thought to have and spread disease. Sometimes this control was directly a result of public health concerns, such as the incarceration of Mary Mallon, or "Typhoid Mary" (McClay 2020). Mallon was under constant surveillance by medical authority figures and her body was a contested site of illness (Hasian 2000).

The construction of disease risk as knowable and preventable has created a new kind of logic about individual risk and responsibility for others' infection. High risk behaviors, such as HIV-positive individuals having unprotected sex with unknowing others (Yee Chan and Reidpath 2003), have become a moral issue and a foci of personal responsibility. This responsibility is framed in a twofold model: first, protecting other people as part of a public health agenda; and second, as a personal responsibility to one's own health. This is a rather modern notion that we have a moral responsibility to maintain our own health. One need only look at the proliferation of fad diets, supplements, and the explosion in popularity of online psychotherapy to see how individuals are compelled to achieve and maintain health and mental health.

In this chapter, I will examine how medical technology in the form of "smart pills" is changing and reinforcing these responsibilities to ourselves and others through the lens of chronic conditions—including HIV, opioid addiction, and severe mental health disorders. I will briefly cover the literature pertaining to smart pills as they relate to HIV/AIDS and opioid addiction but will then turn my gaze to schizophrenia and the smart pill Abilify MyCite (hereafter referred to as MyCite), the first ingestible Bluetooth-enabled pill meant for the surveillance of people with serious mental illness. It has long been established that schizophrenia is not contagious (Hughes 2001). However, people with schizophrenia are socially conditioned to participate in their own care and maintain medication compliance, if indicated and agreed upon by the provider and patient (Treichler and Spaulding 2017). MyCite amounts to technological medical surveillance, which is the modern technologically-enhanced version of the medical surveillance of Mary Mallon (Hasian 2000). Mallon was under constant medical surveillance because of the threat that she posed to others in the form of contagious typhoid fever. This is where the similarities between the surveillance of Mallon and MyCite end: Mallon's typhus was contagious, and she could endanger the lives of people she encountered. Schizophrenia, and the other severe and persistent mental illnesses for which MyCite is prescribed, is not contagious (Hughes 2001).

We can utilize Talcott Parsons's concept of the "sick role" to conceptualize the social responsibility of people with severe mental illness to maintain their medication regimens (Bissell, Traulsen, and Haugbølle 2002; Cockerham 2017). According to Parsons, a sick person has the responsibility to take care of their own health, and if they do so, they are given certain privileges, such as reduced work hours or reduced household or financial responsibilities. The emergence of MyCite and other smart pills seem directly related to Parsonian theory: If one maintains their medication compliance by engaging in voluntary technological surveillance, they will be granted the privileges inherent in the sick role.

In the next sections of this chapter, I will provide a brief background about medical social control and technology, then will discuss the development of smart pills, and will briefly cover how smart pills are used for HIV and opioid addiction. I will then dig deeper into the use of MyCite, and will explore the broader implications of digital pills on the concept of the "deviant body." I will conclude with a discussion about medical surveillance and how it applies to smart pills and will illustrate an arguably dystopian future with the continued development of smart pills.

MEDICAL SOCIAL CONTROL AND TECHNOLOGY

The study of medical social control frequently falls under the larger umbrella of the study of medicalization (Conrad 1992). Early scholars of medicalization and social control anticipated that medical social control would soon supplant other forms of social control (Zola 1972), and while arguably this has not happened, it certainly has expanded (Conrad 1992). In fact, the development of smart pills may have been what Zola (1972) presaged when he said, "It [medicine] is becoming the new repository of truth, the place where absolute and often final judgements are made by supposedly morally neutral and objective experts. And these judgements are made, not in the name of virtue or legitimacy, but in the name of health." According to Conrad (1992), medical social control is often implemented by health professionals, and it is aided by powerful forms of medical technology.

Medical surveillance, as a form of medical social control, is when a certain set of conditions or behaviors come to be seen through a "medical gaze" (Conrad 1992), and physicians lay legitimate claim to all activities concerning the condition. The use of advanced medical technology to help the medical professions engage in medical social control is of the upmost importance. Forms of medical social control include penile implants for male sexual dysfunction (Tiefer 1986) or, more recently, medications for erectile dysfunction (ED) (Potts et al. 2004), hormonal and surgical treatments for people who are transgender (Billings and Urban 1982; Withers 2020), and genetic screening for deafness in infants (Bosteels, Vandenbroeck, and Van Hove 2017). The pairing of medicine and technology can be deadly. The most horrific examples of medical social control involve German physicians' genocidal collaborations with the Nazis, including carrying out the eradication of the "genetically defective" (Conrad 1992). Fortunately, most forms of medical social control are not as diabolical or lethal, but the case of Nazi doctors exemplifies the extreme end of medical social control. In no way am I suggesting that smart pills are equivalent to Nazi purges, but rather wish to illustrate the power that can be generated by the marrying of technology and medicine.

THE LANDSCAPE OF SMART PILLS

Smart pills digitally track, via ingestible Bluetooth technology, whether or not a patient has ingested their prescription medication ("Digital Healthcare 101: What Is Digital Medicine?" 2022). They are composed of three components: an ingestible pill with Bluetooth technology embedded in the tablet; a patch worn on the outside of the body, and a cell phone app. When the 1 mm digital transmitter embedded in the medication interact with stomach chloride, it sends a signal to the patch which subsequently transmits the data to the cell phone application ("Digital Healthcare 101: What Is Digital Medicine?" 2022). The digital signal cannot be activated without contacting these stomach fluids (Chai, Bustamante, et al. 2021; Chai et al. 2017; Chai, Goodman, et al. 2021; Flore 2021). Once the data about the ingestion of the pill reaches the cell phone application, the data is visible to the patient, and if mutually agreeable, is made available to the healthcare provider (or anyone else to whom the patient has granted access to the application). In the case of HIV/AIDS and schizophrenia and other psychotic disorders, digitally tracking medication events is intended to record if the patient has taken their medication and to encourage medication compliance (MBA 2021; Mill et al. 2011). In the case of smart pills and opioids, the digital pill tracking system is intended to record if the patient has taken only the prescribed amount of the opioid (Chai et al. 2017).

Smart pills may very well be the breakthrough pharmaceutical companies were looking for to leapfrog technology into the future. Patents for smart pills currently exist for a diverse range of health phenomena, including mental health, HIV/AIDS, pain control, cardiovascular disease, diabetes, hepatitis C, oncology, tuberculosis, and transplantology (Litvinova et al. 2022). The aim of smart pills is to improve treatment outcomes, increase medication compliance, reduce hospital stays, provide mobile clinical monitoring, have a positive impact on treatment costs, and increase patient safety (Litvinova et al. 2022). Advancement in smart pills is especially focused in the fields of mental health and behavioral modification, such as for schizophrenia, bipolar I disorder, attention deficit and hyperactivity disorder, drug abuse, smoking, pain, insomnia, and many others (Litvinova et al. 2022).

Like Long-Acting Injectable (LAI) depot medications that are intended to improve medication adherence (Okoli et al. 2022), a primary goal of smart pills is to increase medication compliance (Chai, Bustamante, et al. 2021). Non adherence to medication regimens can cause havoc and even death (Chai et al. 2017; Chai, Goodman, et al. 2021). Smart pills are an excellent choice for enabling medication compliance, especially for conditions in which medication adherence tends to be problematic because of the stigma of taking certain medications or the side effect profile of medication (Litvinova et al. 2022; Semahegn et al. 2018). The annual costs of nonadherence range from 100 to 290 billion dollars in the US (Cutler et al. 2018). In addition, 10 percent of hospitalizations among the elderly are due to treatment nonadherence, with a typical nonadherent patient requiring three additional doctor visits per year, resulting in an annual increase of $2,000 in treatment costs (Cutler et al. 2018). For mental health conditions alone, the estimated annual cost per patient of medication nonadherence in the US ranges from $2,512 to $25,920 (Cutler et al. 2018). Clearly, the financial impact of smart pills that increase adherence is enormous, and the adoption of this technology would save health systems and individuals billions.

The first smart pill approved by the FDA in 2017 was Abilify MyCite (Litvinova et al. 2022), an atypical antipsychotic used for the treatment of schizophrenia, schizoaffective disorder, bipolar disorder, and as adjunctive therapy for major depressive disorder (Swartz 2018). MyCite not only tracks drug ingesting patterns, but also mood and activity levels. The four major components of MyCite interact with each other through Bluetooth technology: Aripiprazole (the active medication); an ingestible sensor that transmits information to a patch worn on the rib cage; a mobile app; and an online portal (Litvinova et al. 2022). MyCite is not the only drug equipped with digital sensors to track ingestion. By the end of June 2021, there were 137 digital therapeutic products and 122 personal care products in different stages of development ("Digital Health Trends 2021" 2021). In the next sections of this chapter, I will explore how digital medication is used, often experimentally, in the treatment of HIV/AIDS and opiate addiction, and how these uses demonstrate a form of social control. After providing this overview, I will explore in further detail MyCite and how it is used as a form of medical surveillance and medical social control towards patients with severe and persistent mental illness.

HIV, OPIOIDS, DIGITAL PILLS, AND SOCIAL CONTROL

People living with HIV and AIDS have long been targets for social control and medical surveillance. For example, in Michigan, people living with HIV are required by law to disclose their HIV-positive status to their sexual partners (Hoppe 2013). In the Michigan example, HIV is legally considered a "health threat" (Hoppe 2013) in much the same way as Mary Mallon was considered a threat to others. Medical surveillance like this is a form of social control (Hoppe 2013). There are both formal and informal methods of social control—the formal methods in the case of HIV include epidemiological surveillance such as HIV testing and contact testing, and informal social control is enacted by "third party" phone reports from local residents who accuse people in their community whom they suspect have HIV (Hoppe 2013).

In addition to the concepts of formal and informal social control, there are also forms of positive and negative social control (Fekete, Geaghan, and Druley 2009), which refers to from where the influence comes. Positive social control includes influence from primary network members, and negative social control is enforced behavior change that comes from outside of a patient's primary support network. In the context of HIV, positive social control is associated with more self-care and fewer depressive symptoms, and negative social control is associated with less self-care and more depression (Fekete, Geaghan, and Druley 2009). I argue that smart pills are a form of negative social control, and therefore will lead to less self-care and more depression in all populations.

Stigmatization acts as a social control mechanism for people living with HIV/AIDS (Mill et al. 2011). Stigmatization contributes to inequity for people living with HIV/AIDS, including within the healthcare setting, and includes such practices as shunning, labeling, and disempowerment (Mill et al. 2011). I argue that the use of digital pills further increases stigma because it implies that people living with conditions treated with digital pills such as HIV/AIDS and severe mental illness can't manage their conditions independently. Patients using digital pills may face additional stigma if they choose to not share their private health information, including whether or not they have taken their medication.

Digital pills are used in the administration of HIV PrEP medication, which is prophylactic medication given to people who may have been exposed to the HIV virus. PrEP is effective for preventing HIV after exposure, but it requires consistent compliance (Chai, Goodman, et al. 2021). In addition, smart pills can be used for behavioral interventions, such as if someone is not regularly taking their HIV medication (Chai, Goodman, et al. 2021). Chai, Goodman, et al. (2021) also showed that men who have sex with men and who use substances are willing to engage in smart medication programs and have their medication compliance information transferred to their doctors (Chai, Goodman, et al. 2021).

In addition to their use with HIV/AIDS patients, digital pills are also used for the monitoring of opioid use in the case of severe or post-operative pain. Because opioids are often prescribed in the ER or on an as-needed basis, the dosing schedule is often left up to the patient (Chai et al. 2017; Chai, Goodman, et al. 2021). Chai (Chai et al. 2017) found that a benefit of digital pills for the prescription of opioids is that real-time interventions could be made if doctors detected that a patient was not taking the medication as prescribed. One of the key findings of this study is that clinical trial participants who used the digital pill technology to track the ingestion of opioids after a bone fracture that resulted in the prescription of opioids not only accepted the technology, but many continued to use the digital tracking after the trial period was over (Chai et al. 2017).

MYCITE AND SOCIAL CONTROL

Among physicians, psychiatrists, infectious disease specialists, and public health practitioners are the only doctors charged with managing risk within the community. Psychiatrists and public health officials have historically been given the exclusive right among physicians to take away patients' liberties and freedoms, in the name of protecting the broader community. Psychiatry has a particular and sometimes dark history in which its use of social control may have pushed the boundaries of what is humane or reasonable (Scull 1991). In consideration of this history, it may be no accident that the first smart pill approved by the FDA to monitor drug compliance was designed to treat severe and persistent mental disorders.

The courts are often involved in compulsory psychiatric social control and treatment (Zetterberg, Sjöström, and Markström 2014), but it is foreseeable that drugs like MyCite will eventually replace court involvement, because it puts the control of the deviant psychiatric patient squarely in the hands of the agents of control such as doctors, and perhaps inevitably, other people in positions of power such as employers, parents, and parole officers. MyCite and other still-to-be developed psychiatric smart pills may lead to a diffusion of responsibility for the social control of patients with severe mental illness, shifting responsibility from the court and medical systems to a sociotechnical system comprised of digital technology that is distant from mental health law and practice. This shift away from court involvement to a sociotechnical system may benefit the psychiatric patient. For example, it is often difficult to discriminate how the court makes decisions in terms of compulsory medication, or compulsory psychiatric and/or community treatment (Zetterberg, Sjöström, and Markström 2014). In addition, there are regional and local differences between court decisions, leading to lack of consistency across jurisdictions (Zetterberg, Sjöström, and Markström 2014).

The specter of drugs like MyCite giving physicians increased social control of psychiatric patients may not change the landscape for these patients much: doctors are extremely pressed for time, and the likelihood that doctors will be actively monitoring their patients' MyCite records is low. However, parents, bosses, and other agents of social control may in fact have the time and interest to exert the increased social control that MyCite provides. For example, if a parent or parole officer actively monitors a patient's MyCite records and discovers that the adult patient hasn't been medication compliant, these agents of social control may be able to compel medication adherence by threatening loss of benefits, care, or even, in the case of a parole officer, freedom from incarceration. This increased control could be considered either positive or negative social control (Hoppe 2013). The increased control could either spur the patient into demonstrating better self-care and disorder management or could be negative social control, leading to even less compliance and worsening of depression or other symptoms.

It is important to note that social control and power dynamics already exist between a psychiatric patient and their doctor. Conversation analysis research has considered how pressure is applied by psychiatrists to patients in taking antipsychotic medication (Quirk et al. 2012). The Quirk et al. (2012) study is crucial to understanding the power dynamics between a psychiatric patient and the physician, and MyCite represents an additional level of pressure that psychiatrists can leverage when having discussions about antipsychotics with patients. The impression of shared decision making in psychiatric treatment planning is important to psychiatrists because it mitigates their reputation as merely being agents of social control (Quirk et al. 2012). However, the appearance of MyCite to the psychiatric drug war-chest adds a new wrinkle to the social control of psychiatrists by diffusing the element of control away from the doctor and onto a supposedly neutral sociotechnical system. Ultimately, with traditional medications, the patient can choose whether or not to be medication compliant, but with MyCite, they may lose this autonomy, especially if there are downstream effects or consequences of such monitoring.

ETHICS, TRUTH TELLING, AND MYCITE

Beyond the implications for the doctor-patient relationship and aspects of social control both inside and outside of the medical office, MyCite and other digital pills hold consequences for medical ethics and the ideals of truth telling, trust, and autonomy (Klugman et al. 2018). The perceived benefits of the digital medicine sociotechnical system are continuous and remote monitoring, better disease management, self-tracking, self-management of disease and disorder, and improved medication adherence (Klugman et al. 2018). However, ethical questions arise (Klugman et al. 2018), and these may be especially important in the three cases examined in this chapter of HIV/AIDS, opioid use, and psychiatry. These conditions are often highly stigmatized and patients may have little intrinsic motivation to be honest with their doctors about their adherence to their prescribed medication regimen. In fact, one study showed that 60–80 percent of patients had lied to their doctors (Vogel 2019), most notably about drug use, exercise frequency, and mental health conditions (LSW 2022). MyCite and other digital pills may remove the patient's ability to decide whether they want to tell the truth, although some argue that there exists no "right to lie" (Horton 2022). For ethical reasons, informed consent and a user agreement are critical for a doctor and patient who are about to use MyCite and other digital medication, but these documents raise questions of therapeutic misconception, external influences on decision making, confidentiality and privacy, and device dependability (Klugman et al. 2018). With MyCite, doctors or others can "verify" trust and truth telling.

Swartz (2018) acknowledges that smart pills can improve patient safety and health outcomes, but notes that digital medicine is "underpinned by a singular and inflexible set of values: the belief that quantitative data can provide a coherent model of the world, and the efficacy of bio-data to provide us with ways of acting in it" (Swartz 2018, 65). Swartz (2018) argues that smart pills in the context of serious mental illness are even more ethically tricky than their use in HIV/AIDS treatment, opioid use, and other proposed uses such as diabetes control (Swartz 2018), because of their reification as a supposedly "neutral" technology. MyCite's role as a complex sociotechnical system that involves human actors acting on ethical or unethical premises is lost when patients and agents of social control forget that no technology is neutral.

Mandated treatment and compulsory monitoring are not new nor unique to mental illness. For example, in the United States, convicted sex offenders sometimes have mandated treatment and lifetime monitoring (Walker 2021). Importantly, this mandate and monitoring is done to not only treat the offender, but also to protect the community (Walker 2021). The sex offender model mimics in many ways the sequestering and monitoring of Mary Mallon (McClay 2020). For public health purposes, people with known communicable diseases are often removed from society in order to protect the wider population, such as that which is seen in the case of tuberculosis ("Isolation | Case Management | State TB Prevention & Control Laws | TB Laws & Policies | Resources & Tools | TB | CDC" 2012). A similar form of monitoring and social control was seen in contact tracing (Yuan et al. 2022) and with the concept of social distancing as was seen at the height of the COVID pandemic (Vaterlaus, Spruance, and Patten 2021).

Protecting the safety of others in the community such as in the Mary Mallon case, in HIV/AIDS, or in TB or COVID seems like a noble use of digital pills, but where do we draw the line between ethics and intrusion or social control in situations where the safety of the community at large may not be at risk? Does using digital pills for severe and persistent mental illness pass the "ethics test"? Are we protecting society by enforcing drug compliance? Research has consistently shown that people with severe mental illness, including schizophrenia, schizoaffective disorder, and bipolar disorders, are at increased risk for violent ideation and behavior, but that this risk is increased by comorbid substance use disorders (Roché et al. 2021). One study showed that people with first-episode psychosis present with severe violence in only 0.6 percent of all cases, although committing any violence in the first episode was 34.5 percent (Large and Nielssen 2011). However, severe violence resulting in permanent injury or illness to the victim was uncommon in this population (Large and Nielssen 2011). Alternatively, the risk of self-harming behaviors in persons with schizophrenia spectrum disorders is an even graver problem: in a systematic review, researchers found that deliberate self-harm occurred in up to 69 percent of people with schizophrenia (Lorentzen, Mors, and Kjaer 2022).

CONCLUSION

Digital pills clearly offer a lot of benefit and promise in many areas of healthcare and appear to have benefits for both patients and society at large. However much they have to offer patients, they also represent a form of medical social control (Conrad 1992). Digital pills are poised to control and manage deviance in a way that previous generations of medications are not capable of. For example, gay and bisexual men and IV drug users, who, in the United States are more likely than others to be HIV positive, are both stigmatized groups (Courtenay-Quirk C. et al. 2006; Crandall 1991) and as a result have deviant bodies (Manning 2015) and as such, are ripe for social control (Shipunova 2016). To take the example of digital pills for the management of opioid use, which is currently a huge priority for the United States' social policy (Voon and Kerr 2013), we see again the use of the sociotechnical system of digital medicine acting upon another highly stigmatized group (Wimberly et al. 2022). And of course, the stigma against people with severe and persistent mental illness is well established (Cummings, Lucas, and Druss 2013), and yet again we see digital medicine employed in the management of these deviant and stigmatized bodies.

Taking everything into consideration, protecting the broader community and the patient themselves, digital pills have great promise. However, like the development of all sociotechnical medical systems, unintended consequences and risks may occur (Ash, Berg, and Coiera 2004). For example, digital technology is currently being marketed in the United States for the management of blood sugar levels and insulin delivery in persons with diabetes ("Bionic Pancreas Improves Type 1 Diabetes Management Compared to Standard Insulin Delivery Methods" 2022). Does this use pass the "ethics test" applied to the other cases in this paper? It seems evident and inevitable that digital medicine will permeate every possible medical space in the near future and bioethicists are concerned (Martani et al. 2020). Paranoia and fear about the intrusion of government and business in our bodies is prevalent today in America's communities (Cawkwell and Oshinsky 2015; Sim 2021; "Silencing Debate over Autism" 2007). Are sociotechnical systems like MyCite and other digital pills going to become the newest agents of social control of deviant bodies?

REFERENCES

Ash, Joan S., Marc Berg, and Enrico Coiera. 2004. "Some Unintended Consequences of Information Technology in Health Care: The Nature of Patient Care

Information System-Related Errors." *Journal of the American Medical Informatics Association: JAMIA* 11 (2): 104–12. https://doi.org/10.1197/jamia.M1471.

Billings, Dwight B., and Thomas Urban. 1982. "The Socio-Medical Construction of Transsexualism: An Interpretation and Critique." *Social Problems* 29 (3): 266–82. https://doi.org/10.2307/800159.

"Bionic Pancreas Improves Type 1 Diabetes Management Compared to Standard Insulin Delivery Methods." 2022. National Institutes of Health (NIH). September 28, 2022. https://www.nih.gov/news-events/news-releases/bionic-pancreas-improves-type-1-diabetes-management-compared-standard-insulin-delivery-methods.

Bissell, Paul, Janine Morgall Traulsen, and Lotte Stig Haugbølle. 2002. "Sociological Theory and Pharmacy Practice Research: (2) An Introduction to Functionalist Sociology: Talcott Parsons' Concept of the 'Sick Role.'" *International Journal of Pharmacy Practice* 10 (1): 60–68. https://doi.org/10.1111/j.20427174.2002.tb00589.x.

Bosteels, Sigrid, Michel Vandenbroeck, and Geert Van Hove. 2017. "Saving Deaf Children? Screening for Hearing Loss as a Public-Interest Case." *Journal of Bioethical Inquiry* 14 (1): 109–21. https://doi.org/10.1007/s11673-016-9752-y.

Cawkwell, Philip B., and David Oshinsky. 2015. "Childhood Vaccination Requirements: Lessons from History, Mississippi, and a Path Forward." *Vaccine* 33 (43): 5884–87. https://doi.org/10.1016/j.vaccine.2015.08.087.

Chai, Peter R., Maria J. Bustamante, Georgia Goodman, Yassir Mohamed, Jesse Najarro, Matthew C. Sullivan, Jose Castillo-Mancilla, et al. 2021. "A Brief Training Program to Support the Use of a Digital Pill System for Medication Adherence: Pilot Descriptive Study." *JMIR Formative Research* 5 (4): e26213. https://doi.org/10.2196/26213.

Chai, Peter R., Stephanie Carreiro, Brendan J. Innes, Brittany Chapman, Kristin L. Schreiber, Robert R. Edwards, Adam W. Carrico, and Edward W. Boyer. 2017. "Oxycodone Ingestion Patterns in Acute Fracture Pain With Digital Pills:" *Anesthesia & Analgesia* 125 (6): 2105–12. https://doi.org/10.1213/ANE.0000000000002574.

Chai, Peter R., Georgia Goodman, Majo Bustamante, Lizette Mendez, Yassir Mohamed, Kenneth H. Mayer, Edward W. Boyer, Rochelle K. Rosen, and Conall O'Cleirigh. 2021. "Design and Delivery of Real-Time Adherence Data to Men Who Have Sex with Men Using Antiretroviral Pre-Exposure Prophylaxis via an Ingestible Electronic Sensor." *AIDS & Behavior* 25 (6): 1661–74. https://doi.org/10.1007/s10461-020-03082-y.

Cockerham, William C. 2017. *Medical Sociology*. 14th edition. New York, NY: Routledge.

Conrad, Peter. 1992. "Medicalization and Social Control." *Annual Review of Sociology* 18: 209–32.

Courtenay-Quirk C., R. J. Wolitski, J. T. Parsons, and C. A. Gómez. 2006. "Is HIV/AIDS Stigma Dividing the Gay Community? Perceptions of HIV-Positive Men Who Have Sex with Men." *AIDS Education & Prevention* 18 (1): 56–67. https://doi.org/10.1521/aeap.2006.18.1.56.

Crandall, Christian S. 1991. "Multiple Stigma and AIDS: Illness Stigma and Attitudes Toward Homosexuals and IV Drug Users in AIDS-Related Stigmatization." *Journal of Community & Applied Social Psychology* 1 (2): 165–72. https://doi.org/10.1002/casp.2450010210.

Cummings, Janet R., Stephen M. Lucas, and Benjamin G. Druss. 2013. "Addressing Public Stigma and Disparities Among Persons With Mental Illness: The Role of Federal Policy." *American Journal of Public Health* 103 (5): 781–85.

Cutler, Rachelle Louise, Fernando Fernandez-Llimos, Michael Frommer, Charlie Benrimoj, and Victoria Garcia-Cardenas. 2018. "Economic Impact of Medication Non-Adherence by Disease Groups: A Systematic Review." *BMJ Open* 8 (1): e016982. https://doi.org/10.1136/bmjopen-2017016982.

"Digital Health Trends 2021." 2021. https://www.iqvia.com/insights/the-iqvia-institute/reports/digital-health-trends-2021.

"Digital Healthcare 101: What Is Digital Medicine?" 2022. *MDBriefCase* (blog). May 10, 2022. https://www.mdbriefcase.com/digital-healthcare-101-what-is-digital-medicine/.

Fekete, Erin, Thomas R. Geaghan, and Jennifer Ann Druley. 2009. "Affective and Behavioural Reactions to Positive and Negative Health-Related Social Control in HIV+ Men." *Psychology & Health* 24 (5): 501–15. https://doi.org/10.1080/08870440801894674.

Flore, Jacinthe. 2021. "Ingestible Sensors, Data, and Pharmaceuticals: Subjectivity in the Era of Digital Mental Health." *New Media & Society* 23 (7): 2034–51. https://doi.org/10.1177/1461444820931024.

Hasian, Marouf A. 2000. "Power, Medical Knowledge, and the Rhetorical Invention of 'Typhoid Mary.'" *Journal of Medical Humanities* 21 (3): 123–39. https://doi.org/10.1023/A:1009074619421.

Hoppe, Trevor. 2013. "Controlling Sex in the Name of 'Public Health': Social Control and Michigan HIV Law." *Social Problems* 60 (1): 27–49. https://doi.org/10.1525/sp.2013.60.1.27.

Horton, Richard. 2022. "Offline: There Is No Right to Lie." *The Lancet* 399 (10327): 778. https://doi.org/10.1016/S0140-6736(22)003701.

Hughes, William. 2001. "Schizophrenia Is Not Contagious | Psychiatric Services." 2001. https://ps-psychiatryonline-org.proxy.lib.pdx.edu/doi/full/10.1176/appi.ps.52.3.384.

"Isolation | Case Management | State TB Prevention & Control Laws | TB Laws & Policies | Resources & Tools | TB | CDC." 2012. https://www.cdc.gov/tb/programs/laws/menu/isolation.htm.

Klugman, Craig M., Laura B. Dunn, Jack Schwartz, and I. Glenn Cohen. 2018. "The Ethics of Smart Pills and Self-Acting Devices: Autonomy, Truth-Telling, and Trust at the Dawn of Digital Medicine." *American Journal of Bioethics* 18 (9): 38–47. https://doi.org/10.1080/15265161.2018.1498933.

Large, Matthew M., and Olav Nielssen. 2011. "Violence in First-Episode Psychosis: A Systematic Review and Meta-Analysis." *Schizophrenia Research* 125 (2): 209–20. https://doi.org/10.1016/j.schres.2010.11.026.

Litvinova, Olena, Elisabeth Klager, Nikolay T. Tzvetkov, Oliver Kimberger, Maria Kletecka-Pulker, Harald Willschke, and Atanas G. Atanasov. 2022. "Digital Pills with Ingestible Sensors: Patent Landscape Analysis." *Pharmaceuticals* 15 (8): 1025. https://doi.org/10.3390/ph15081025.

Lorentzen, E., O. Mors, and J. N. Kjaer. 2022. "The Prevalence of Self-Harm Behavior in Schizophrenia Spectrum Disorders: A Systematic Review and Meta-Analysis." *European Psychiatry* 65 (S1): S766. https://doi.org/10.1192/j.eurpsy.2022.1978.

Manning, Taylor C. 2015. "Obstacles, Transitions, & Perspectives: An In-Depth Look at the Spectacle of Deviant Bodies." M.A. diss., East Tennessee State University. https://www.proquest.com/docview/1846960940/abstract/E95018398934607PQ/1.

Martani, Andrea, Darryl Geneviève Lester, Christopher Poppe, Carlo Casonato, and Tenzin Wangmo. 2020. "Digital Pills: A Scoping Review of the Empirical Literature and Analysis of the Ethical Aspects." *BMC Medical Ethics* 21: 1–13. https://doi.org/10.1186/s12910-019-0443-1.

McClay, B. D. 2020. "Learning from Typhoid Mary." *The Hedgehog Review* 22 (2): 16–20.

Mill, Judy, Nancy Edwards, Randy Jackson, Lynne MacLean, and Jean Chaw-Kant. 2011. "Stigmatization as a Social Control Mechanism for Persons Living with HIV and AIDS." https://doi.org/10.1177/1049732310375436.

Newton, David. 2020. "Germ Theory—Gale In Context: Environmental Studies." 2020. https://go-gale-com.proxy.lib.pdx.edu/ps/i.do?p=GRNR&u=s1185784&id=GALE|CX7947900124&v=2.1&it=r.

Norreel, Jean-Chretien, PhD. 2021. "Are Smart Pills the Future of Medication Adherence?" *Digital Health Central* (blog). September 14, 2021. https://digitalhealthcentral.com/2021/09/14/smart-pill/.

Okoli, Chizimuzo T.C., Amani Kappi, Tianyi Wang, Andrew Makowski, and Andrew T. Cooley. 2022. "The Effect of Long-Acting Injectable Antipsychotic Medications Compared with Oral Antipsychotic Medications among People with Schizophrenia: A Systematic Review and Meta-Analysis." *International Journal of Mental Health Nursing* 31 (3): 469–535. https://doi.org/10.1111/inm.12964.

Potts, Annie, Victoria Grace, Nicola Gavey, and Tiina Vares. 2004. "'Viagra Stories': Challenging 'Erectile Dysfunction.'" *Social Science & Medicine* 59 (3): 489–99. https://doi.org/10.1016/j.socscimed.2003.06.001.

Quirk, Alan, Rob Chaplin, Paul Lelliott, and Clive Seale. 2012. "How Pressure Is Applied in Shared Decisions about Antipsychotic Medication: A Conversation Analytic Study of Psychiatric Outpatient Consultations: CA of Psychiatric Outpatient Consultations." *Sociology of Health & Illness* 34 (1): 95–113. https://doi.org/10.1111/j.14679566.2011.01363.x.

Roché, Matthew W., Douglas J. Boyle, Chia-Cherng Cheng, Jill Del Pozzo, Lindsay Cherneski, Joe Pascarella, Alicia Lukachko, and Steven M. Silverstein. 2021. "Prevalence and Risk of Violent Ideation and Behavior in Serious Mental Illnesses: An Analysis of 63,572 Patient Records." *Journal of Interpersonal Violence* 36 (5–6): 2732–52. https://doi.org/10.1177/0886260518759976.

Scull, Andrew. 1991. "Psychiatry and Social Control in the Nineteenth and Twentieth Centuries." *History of Psychiatry* 2 (6): 149–69. https://doi.org/10.1177/0957154X9100200603.

Semahegn, Agumasie, Kwasi Torpey, Abubakar Manu, Nega Assefa, Gezahegn Tesfaye, and Augustine Ankomah. 2018. "Psychotropic Medication Non-Adherence and Associated Factors among Adult Patients with Major Psychiatric Disorders: A Protocol for a Systematic Review." *Systematic Reviews* 7. https://doi.org/10.1186/s13643-018-0676-y.

Shipunova, Tatyana. 2016. "Features of the Social Control of Deviance." *Sociological Research* 55 (1): 31–44. https://doi.org/10.1080/10610154.2016.1184067.

"Silencing Debate over Autism." 2007. *Nature Neuroscience* 10 (5): 531. https://doi.org/10.1038/nn0507531.

Sim, Shaun. 2021. "Should Businesses Mandate That Staff Get the Covid Vaccine? Employers Seek a Safe Return to Work, but Forcing the Issue May Not Be Feasible." https://go-gale-com.proxy.lib.pdx.edu/ps/i.do?p=ITBC&u=s1185784&id=GALE%7CA648347946&v=2.1&it=r.

Swartz, Anna K. 2018. "Smart Pills for Psychosis: The Tricky Ethical Challenges of Digital Medicine for Serious Mental Illness." *American Journal of Bioethics* 18 (9): 65–67. https://doi.org/10.1080/15265161.2018.1498948.

Tiefer, Leonore. 1986. "In Pursuit of the Perfect Penis: 'The Medicalization of Male Sexuality.'" *The American Behavioral Scientist* 29 (5): 579–99.

Treichler, Emily B. H., and William D. Spaulding. 2017. "Beyond Shared Decision-Making: Collaboration in the Age of Recovery from Serious Mental Illness." *American Journal of Orthopsychiatry* 87 (5): 567–74. https://doi.org/10.1037/ort0000256.

Vaterlaus, J. Mitchell, Lori A. Spruance, and Emily V. Patten. 2021. "COVID-19 Pandemic and Social Distancing in the United States: A Mixed-Methods Study on Lived Experiences and Well-Being." *The Social Science Journal*: 1–13. https://doi.org/10.1080/03623319.2020.1852856.

Vogel, Lauren. 2019. "Why Do Patients Often Lie to Their Doctors?" *CMAJ: Canadian Medical Association Journal* 191 (4): E115. https://doi.org/10.1503/cmaj.1095705.

Voon, Pauline, and Thomas Kerr. 2013. "'Nonmedical' Prescription Opioid Use in North America: A Call for Priority Action." *Substance Abuse Treatment, Prevention, and Policy* 8 (1): 39. https://doi.org/10.1186/1747597X-839.

Walker, Andrea M. 2021. "A Delicate Dance: Ethical and Systemic Issues in Providing Community-Based Sex Offender Treatment." *Sexual Abuse* 33 (7): 769–92. https://doi.org/10.1177/1079063220965946.

Wimberly, Alexandra S., Ryan Petros, Paul Sacco, Maura Tennor, Shawna Murray-Browne, and Loraine Arikat. 2022. "Factors That Contribute to Stigma toward Opioid Users among Social Work Students." *Journal of Social Work Practice in the Addictions*: 1–12. https://doi.org/10.1080/1533256X.2022.2103982.

Withers, Robert. 2020. "Transgender Medicalization and the Attempt to Evade Psychological Distress." *Journal of Analytical Psychology* 65 (5): 865–89. https://doi.org/10.1111/14685922.12641.

Yasgur, Batya Swift. 2022. "An Uncomfortable Truth: Why Patients Lie to Their Physicians." MPR. June 13, 2022. https://www.empr.com/home/features/an-uncomfortable-truth-why-patients-lie-to-their-physicians/.

Yee Chan, Kit, and Daniel D Reidpath. 2003. "'Typhoid Mary' and 'HIV Jane': Responsibility, Agency and Disease Prevention." *Reproductive Health Matters* 11 (22): 40–50. https://doi.org/10.1016/S0968-8080(03)022912.

Yuan, Xiaojun, DeeDee Bennett Gayle, Yvonne Dadson, and Ellie Jung. 2022. "Perception and Use of COVID Contact Tracing Mobile Applications in New York State (NYS)." *Proceedings of the Association for Information Science and Technology* 59 (1): 845–47. https://doi.org/10.1002/pra2.746.

Zetterberg, Liv, Stefan Sjöström, and Urban Markström. 2014. "The Compliant Court—Procedural Fairness and Social Control in Compulsory Community Care." *International Journal of Law and Psychiatry* 37 (6): 543–50. https://doi.org/10.1016/j.ijlp.2014.02.027.

Zola, Irving Kenneth. 1972. "Medicine as an Institution of Social Control." *The Sociological Review* 20 (4): 487–504. https://doi.org/10.1111/j.1467954X.1972.tb00220.x.

Index

About the Contributors

Kathryn Burrows is an assistant professor of sociology at Madonna University and an independent scholar. She received her PhD in sociology from Portland State University and she attended Rutgers University for all her coursework and the majority of the dissertation research. Her research interests are broad, spanning across the spectrum of medical sociology and concepts of normality, including disability studies and medical technology. She is particularly interested in concepts of social control and deviance as it relates to medical technology and is currently working on an empirical paper about users of Abilify MyCite. Previous work includes substantial investigations into the social meanings of deafness and D/deaf technologies and research about the social construction of bipolar disorder "epidemics" and the gender stereotypes of genital cancer survivors.

Misria Shaik Ali is currently assistant professor, School of Arts and Design, Woxsen University, Hyderabad. She holds a PhD in Science and Technology Studies and her dissertation is titled "Becoming Irradiated: The Epistemic Politics of Neglect along India's Nuclear Fuel Cycle." Her research advances the field of Critical Nuclear Studies by putting Science and Technology Studies, Feminist Science Studies, Postcolonial Studies, Agnotology, Sensory Studies, Eco-crip theory, and Nuclear Studies in conversation with one another. She also works on the ongoing genocide of Muslims in/of India and her research and writing address Muslim alterity in India with a focus on religious studies, alterity studies, and violence studies. Her research and writings are published in academic publication platforms like *Tapuya Magazine*, *RSA Journal*, Centre for 21st Century blog, and *Seminar Magazine*, and in newspapers like Maktoob Media, TwoCircles.net, FirstPost, and *Outlook Magazine* among others.

Amber Nicole Brooks is an associate professor of English at Georgia State University and a PhD candidate at Georgia Institute of Technology, in an interdisciplinary History and Sociology program. Brooks' current research investigates the historical, social, and cultural dimensions of contraceptive technologies, with a focus on situational and discourse analysis. Her dissertation research focuses on the IUD in the U.S., from menstrual suppression to access post-Dobbs. Her work in various genres has appeared in *Peitho: Journal of the Coalition of Feminist Scholars in the History of Rhetoric and Composition*, *The Arkansas Review*, *The Chattahoochee Review*, *The Southeastern Review*, *The Collagist*, *The Rumpus*, and *ArtsATL*.

Indira Chakravarthi is a public health researcher and teacher based in Delhi, India. She has graduate training in biochemistry and completed her doctoral dissertation on diffusion of medical technology in India. Her areas of interest and study are: technology, medicine, and health; healthcare systems and health policy. Her research and publications have covered issues such as diffusion, procurement, policies and regulation of medical technology in India, specific technologies such as vaccination and assisted reproductive technologies; healthcare systems issues such as corporatization and commercialization, and universal health care; and social determinants of health. She is currently (2023–2024) a guest faculty in the Public Health program at Dr. B.R. Ambedkar University, Delhi.

Alan Hawk has been Collections Manager of the Historical Collections of the National Museum of Health and Medicine since 1987. He is responsible for care and development of a 15,000-artifact collection documenting the history of medical technology, with an emphasis on military medicine. In 2017, he retired from the U.S. Navy Reserve as a Senior Chief Petty Officer, with a 30-year career that included one deployment to Afghanistan in 2009 as well as previous service in the 1/115th Infantry in the Maryland Army National Guard. Prior to his present position, he served as Assistant Historic Preservation Planner for the City of Wilmington, Delaware, and as a Historical Consultant for the Methodist Action Program. He also assisted in the computerization project of the National Register of Historic Places for the National Park Service. He received his bachelor's degree in history from the University of Delaware in 1983. He is married and has two adult children.

Danielle Kabella received a PhD in Human and Social Dimension of Science and Technology at Arizona State University's School for the Future of Innovation. Their doctoral research offers an ethnographic study that makes visible alternative strategies Chicanx communities use to articulate place-based drug recovery futures in New Mexico. Dr. Kabella recently joined UCSF as an Opioid Industry Documents Archive (OIDA) postdoctoral fellow, funded through the UCSF Center for Tobacco Control Research and

Education (CTCRE) and working with Drs. Knight and Apollonia. They are conducting research that enables scrutiny and analysis of the manifestation of place and race in the wider context of corporate and regulatory practice. Taking seriously the methodological approach of *archiving* as a human right, they are exploring community-led knowledge production strategies in leveraging OIDA.

Jenny Kennedy is associate professor in media and commuication at RMIT University, Australia. She is an associate investigator in the ARC Centre of Excellence for Automated Decision-Making and Society (ADM+S) and is a core member of the Digital Ethnography Research Centre (DERC). Her research charts barriers to digital inclusion against the context of rapid evolutions in digital infrastructures, smart devices, artificial intelligence, and automated decision-making. Jenny's most recent coauthored books include *Digital Domesticity: Media, Materiality and Home Life* (2020) and *The Smart Wife: Why Alexa, Siri and Other Smart Home Devices Need a Feminist Reboot* (2020).

Ankita Mukherjee is qualitative researcher at the George Institute for Global Health, India. She has extensive experience of using qualitative methods in health services research and program evaluation. In her current role she is part of an interdisciplinary team that is working on a multi-site community-based randomized control trial, testing digital health interventions to address mental disorders in India. In the past she has done research assignments in diverse areas including sexual and reproductive health, health financing schemes, and medical technology. Her doctoral dissertation was on adoption and diffusion of medical technologies in India. Ankita holds a PhD degree in Social Medicine and Community Health from Jawaharlal Nehru University, New Delhi. Her research interests include health systems and policy research, implementation research, and approaches to program evaluation.

Anna Gonzalez Suero holds a PhD in Art from Goldsmiths, University of London. As an artistic researcher, she works with autoethnography to explore the aesthetic dimensions of medico-technical images appearing on screens and as models, with a focus on the visual and material cultures of gynecology and obstetrics. Gonzalez Suero works on challenging fundamental ideas around images with medical origins by engaging different materials and media, including drawing, video, text, and collage. Recently, she published an autoethnographic essay, "The Foetus Phallus Studio," in the edited volume *Performing the Penis: Phalluses in 21st Century Cultures* (2022).

Rowan Wilken is associate professor in Media and Communication, and an associate investigator in the Australian Research Council Centre of Excellence for Automated Decision-Making and Society, at RMIT University, Melbourne, Australia. Rowan researches mobile and location-based media, machine vision, the history of vehicle automation and navigation, everyday data cultures, and the enduring significance of residual media and communication technologies. He is the coauthor (with Ingrid Richardson) of *Bodies and Mobile Media* (2023), coauthor (with Jean Burgess, Kath Albury, and Anthony McCosker) of *Everyday Data Cultures* (2022), coauthor (with Anthony McCosker) of *Automating Vision: The Social Impact of the New Camera Consciousness* (2020), author of *Cultural Economies of Locative Media* (2019), coeditor (with Gerard Goggin and Heather A. Horst) of *Location Technologies in International Context* (2019), coeditor (with Justin Clemens) of *The Afterlives of Georges Perec* (2017), coeditor (with Gerard Goggin) of *Locative Media* (2014) and *Mobile Technology and Place* (2012), and author of *Teletechnologies, Place, and Community* (2011).